Improving
Upper Body Control

An Approach to Assessment and Treatment of Tonal Dysfunction

by Regi Boehme, O.T.R.

Illustrations by John Boehme

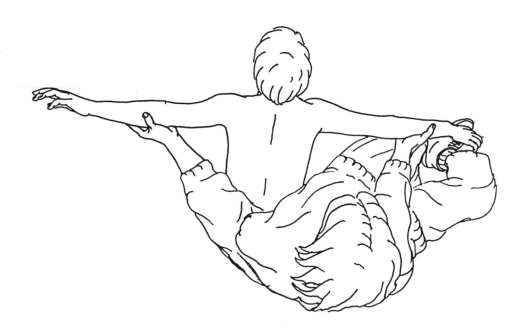

Therapy Skill Builders
A division of
Communication Skill Builders
3830 E. Bellevue/P.O. Box 42050
Tucson, Arizona 85733/(602) 323-7500

Text © 1988 by Regi Boehme
Illustrations © 1988 by John Boehme

Printed and Published 1988 by:

Therapy Skill Builders
A division of
Communication Skill Builders
3830 E. Bellevue/P.O. Box 42050
Tucson, Arizona 85733/(602) 323-7500

ISBN 0-88450-262-7   Catalog No. 4137

        10 9 8 7 6
Printed in the United States of America

About the Author

Regi Boehme graduated from Western Michigan University with a B.S. degree in occupational therapy. She is a certified occupational therapy instructor in neurodevelopmental treatment and has lectured internationally on topics related to neurological dysfunction. Her Milwaukee-based treatment clinic provides assessment, treatment, and consultation services for both pediatric and adult patients from around the world.

Regi has spent her life being curious. Her experiences with those challenged by gravity have led to this book. Her focus on teaching has led her to the realization that the therapy professions are filled with gifted people who are also curious.

They, too, have led to this book.

About the Illustrator

John Boehme graduated from St. Norberts College with a BS degree in psychology. His avocation of stained glass designing has led to his "love of line" which is expressed in his illustrations. He is the executive director of Boehme Workshops, offering state-of-the-art continuing education opportunities for individuals involved in the care of children with neurological dysfunction.

Acknowledgments

This book has been an interesting journey. I met significant people on the way: I would like to thank them for their insights.

Dr. Ruth Jansen,
who introduced me to children

Barbara Cupps, P.T.,
who introduced me to neurodevelopmental treatment

Dr. Karel and Berta Bobath,
for their living concept of neurodevelopmental treatment

Lois Bly, P.T.,
for her concrete analysis of movement

John Barnes, P.T.,
for broadening my perspective on touch

My children, Holly and Peter,
who taught me how to love and relate to the young,
the young at heart, and those searching for their youth

Mary Ellen Boehme,
who edited, searched for drawings, and established
a strong relationship with a Xerox machine

My patients and the participants in my seminars
who challenged, stimulated, and trusted me

My parents and brother,
who provided support from many perspectives

. . . and John Boehme,
my illustrator, my partner, my soul mate

Preface

This book will help you assess and treat patients with neurological impairment resulting in dysfunctional or abnormal muscle tone.

The material concentrates on achieving upper extremity function for personal autonomy. However, because the upper extremities work in synchrony with the rest of the body, it covers significant aspects of whole body movement as well. Thus, though the book is written by an occupational therapist, physical therapists and speech pathologists will find the information applicable to gait and respiration.

This information can be applied to patients of any age or size. The illustrations alternate the use of small and large bodies so you can generalize your visualizations.

The intervention strategies presented reflect a strong neurodevelopmental treatment orientation. However, the analysis of component parts of movement and the review of significant aspects of normal and abnormal development have evolved from the integration of anatomical and kinesiological perspectives. Our kinesiology illustrations are intended to help you visualize the position of the muscle and the related skeletal parts. As you provide treatment, these visual images will guide the location and direction of your touch.

Treating the patient who has had a neurological injury is a challenge because we cannot remove the central nervous system lesion. The premise of the neurodevelopmental treatment approach is that we can change function by giving the sensorimotor system more appropriate cues. When we work with an immature central nervous system, we are guiding the original developmental process. When we work with a matured system, our focus is on retraining. In both cases, the therapist's sensorimotor system relates to and modifies the sensorimotor system of the patient. It becomes a graceful and fluid interaction.

Therapy is like good art and science. It is often a matter of taking advantage of the fortuitous "accident." Enjoy.

Contents

Chapter 1 **Touch** 1
   Inhibition and Facilitation 3
   Key Points of Control 4
   Grading Your Input 6
       Sustained Light Pressure 6
       Sustained Deep Pressure 7
       Intermittent Touch 7
   Treatment with Movement—Slow Movement 8
       Fast Movement 8
   Treatment with Compression and Traction 9
       Sustained Joint Traction 10
       Sustained Joint Compression 12
       Intermittent Compression 13
       Other Forms of Tapping 14
       The Concept of Assessment 16
       The Concept of Carryover 17
       The Concept of Treatment 17
   References 18

Chapter 2 **The Role of the Shoulder Girdle in Posture and Movement** 19
   Prologue 19
   The Value of Symmetry 20
   Symmetrical Control of Posture 20
   Unilateral Control of Posture 24
   Diagonal Control 25
   Dynamic Sitting 26

Chapter 3 **Analysis and Treatment for Horizontal Reach** 27
   Movements of the Arm in a Horizontal Plane 27
       Horizontal Humeral Abduction 27
       Horizontal Humeral Adduction 43
   Summary 58
   References 58

Chapter 4 **Analysis and Treatment for Wide-Range Reach** 59
   Movements of the Arm Above the Head 59
       Humeral Flexion 59
   Summary 86
   References 86

Chapter 5 **Treatment of Basic Hand Function** 87
   The Functional Perspective 87
       Forearm Rotation 88
       The Wrist 95
       The Hand 98
       Release 116
   Summary 117
   References 118

Chapter 6 **Digital Manipulation** 119
               Introduction 119
               Radial-Digital Grasp 119
               Three-Jawed Chuck 120
               Pinch 121
               Reciprocal Patterns of Movement 123
               Sequential Patterns of Movement 124
               Complex Patterns of Movement 126
               References 127

Appendixes
Appendix A: Current Trends in Upper Extremity Splinting 131
Appendix B: Casting to Improve Upper Extremity Function 165
Appendix C: A Kinesiological Analysis of Dynamic Sitting 189

CHAPTER 1

Touch

I have been the recipient and victim of many "therapeutic" hands, many of them not at all therapeutic. The touch of most medical people, for example, is fairly annoying. They vacillate between a fingertip touch and an abrupt grip and torque which creates massive tissue guarding. "Did that hurt?" My description of how to touch patients and communicate with them is based partially on my personal experiences.

I had surgery a few years ago to correct a problem created by the effects of polio. The surgery altered the position of the left foot in relationship to the leg and dramatically changed my posture in standing. The new foot position brought my knee out of thirty degrees of hyperextension, into neutral. It reduced my severe anterior pelvic tilt and shoulder girdle retraction. After surgery I looked great, but I could not walk. I could not initiate gait with the new alignment. I could not even shift my weight. Traditional exercises and gait training did not solve my problem.

With the help of a therapist certified in neurodevelopmental treatment, I learned to move in space. We both learned a great deal about the impact of therapy on the whole patient. For example, I spent a great part of my treatment session asking the therapist what she was doing: "Talk to me back there!" She quietly worked behind me, stimulating weight shifting, stepping, and gait. She had a gentle touch and yet I felt as if I were being pushed and pulled around. The smallest weight shift, when unexpected, frightened me. I guarded or held against it. I often felt agitated during therapy. We tried working in front of a mirror where we could see each other and I could see myself. However, emotionally I could not tolerate the image of an erect body. It did not match my body image. I could not accept and use unfamiliar movements with the unfamiliar mirror image.

My movements in space quickly improved. Nevertheless it took some time for my proprioceptive senses to catch up with the new movements. I would lean over to shut the car door, and I would fall out of the car. The length of my arm changed with the new alignment of my shoulders. I would try to put a cup of coffee on the kitchen table, but instead it would land on the floor. Furthermore, I lost my penmanship. I could not sign my name for well over two weeks. My creditors were up in arms!

Yet another interesting phenomenon took place. I could feel and initiate a better pattern in gait during therapy, but within a few hours, I could no longer use the pattern. I lost the feeling of the movement. I could no longer initiate the movement because I could not visualize it. I felt I did not yet own the movement.

I have learned to slow down and talk with my patients. I tell them what I am going to do and what they might expect to happen. I talk with all of my patients, whether they are adults or infants. I grade my handling according to the patients' emotional responses as well as how their bodies respond. I earn their trust and try not to abuse it. We share control over the session. We work as a team rather than struggle against each other. They agree to work hard and I agree to be a caring and gentle person. It appears to be a reasonable trade-off.

It is sometimes hard to reason and trade off with young children. They, like the adults, are often afraid of new movement patterns. Occasionally, the children cry during therapy. They become angry and frustrated. They do not understand that my hands are there to help, rather than intrude. Sometimes I treat them in their parents' laps where they feel safe. This does not always work. I offer them toys that can be used in many different ways, so they can experience success rather than failure. I encourage children to be imaginative. I stimulate their ability to visualize movement: "Today you are the airplane and I am the cloud." I give them ample periods of time to move without my hands on them.

As we treat patients, we gather information. We analyze their responses to our handling input by observing their movement. The change in their ability to move may or may not be what we predicted, but it provides us with the opportunity to gather more information. We utilize trial and error to collect information. The sensory input we offer a patient undergoes continual modification during this ongoing assessment process. This is a spontaneous process. As we receive and interpret information about a patient's movement, we transmit sensorimotor data back to the patient and wait for a response. As the patient is responding, we are modifying the input from our hands. With an intimate knowledge of normal movement dynamics and a variety of handling possibilities, the process of treatment becomes a graceful, fluid interaction.

This chapter will describe several ways of modifying sensorimotor input to obtain predictable changes in the patient's motor repertoire. As you read the chapter, I encourage you to therapeutically touch and handle as many able-bodied people as possible. This is probably not the worst suggestion you have ever received. You will find that every individual body feels slightly different. Muscle tone varies from person to person. Each body's approach to movement has unique qualities. Each person's level of comfort with touching varies. You can learn a great deal by practicing handling on others, because you can take your time and receive feedback about your perceptions. Once you become comfortable with the many different ways of modifying sensory information, you will find yourself changing your pressure, speed, and hand placement naturally during your treatment sessions. Before you begin, a review of terminology is in order.

Inhibition and Facilitation

Inhibition is the process of intervention that reduces dysfunctional muscle tone. Setting specific techniques aside for the moment, inhibition reduces the intensity of spasticity, making greater range and variety of movement possible. Inhibition reduces the influence of fluctuating muscle tone, making the control of mid- or small-range movements possible. Inhibition is not used with hypotonicity.

On the other hand, *facilitation* is the process of intervention which uses the improved muscle tone in goal-directed activity. The patient is active, and the therapist is guiding the activity. Facilitation makes movement easier. The movement is guided by your hands. You can stop the movement in midstream (Figure 1). Any time your hands stop, the patient's movements will also stop.

Inhibition is used with facilitation. They are accomplished simultaneously, with the least amount of physical intrusion. As you use techniques that inhibit dysfunctional tone, the patient makes more efficient movement adaptations. This happens spontaneously because your patients are actively involved in functional movement and automatic postural reactions while your hands treat them. The concept of inhibition and facilitation was first described by Berta and Dr. Karel Bobath, the pioneers in neurodevelopmental treatment.

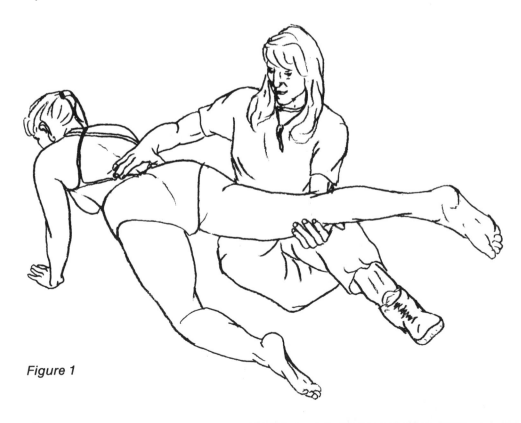

Figure 1

Key Points of Control

The places where we make physical contact with the patient are referred to as key points of control (Bobath 1980). We can key-point with our hands and any other parts of our body (Figure 2). We can key-point with our whole hand or fingertips. We can use therapy equipment or any surface as a key point of control (Figure 3).

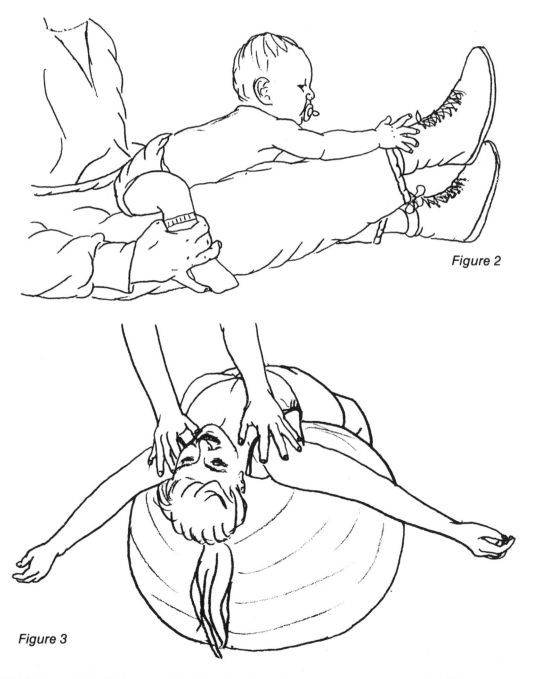

Figure 2

Figure 3

Key points of control near the source of the problem are referred to as proximal. Proximal can also mean close to the head, torso, or large joints. In any event, proximal key points allow the handler the option of taking control of the patient's body during difficult movements (Figure 4).

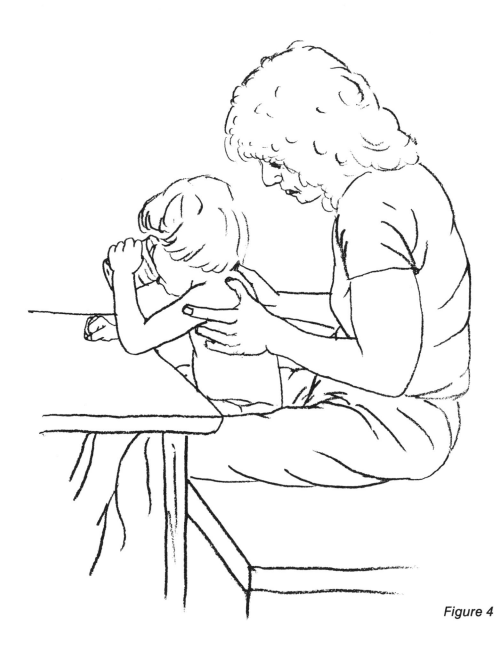

Figure 4

Key points of control away from the problem source are referred to as distal. Hand placement on the extremities or away from the torso is also considered distal. With distal key points of control, the therapist is less able to control the patient's whole body response (Figure 5). When hand placement is at a distance from the problem, the patient will perform the majority of the work. The ultimate goal during therapy is to provide the least amount of intervention, as far as possible from the problem.

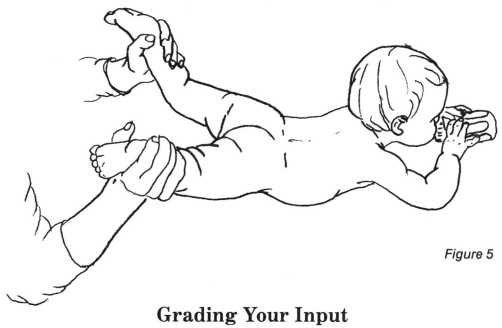

Figure 5

Grading Your Input

When I treat a patient, I respond to what I see and feel. I concentrate on eliminating the "background noise" coming from my own body, and focus on synchronizing myself with the patient's body. I trust my hands and grade my touch.

SUSTAINED LIGHT PRESSURE

I always begin with light touch. Light, nonintrusive touch can be felt through the hair and surface of the skin. With light touch you will not be able to palpate muscle and joint.

By placing the whole hand gently, anywhere on the patient, in a nonintrusive way, the patient will relax under your touch. You will gain important information about how movement is initiated, how the patient is attempting to control posture against gravity for independent function, and how compensation is made for the limited movement repertoire. You can develop a sense of the subtle central nervous system problems, signs that one might not observe visually. Your hands follow the movement and gently intervene by resisting the abnormal responses, without taking away the patient's active control. You make the small adjustments necessary to allow the patient to continue to function. The goal is to create movement that is easier and more fluid rather than simply concentrating on achieving "normal" movement. As the patient engages in functional movement, light touch guides rather than controls. The emphasis is on facilitation with subtle, nonintrusive inhibition.

SUSTAINED DEEP PRESSURE

When a patient is continually bound by the same nonfunctional movement patterns, a gradual increase in your pressure is appropriate. With deep pressure you can feel the muscles and as you add more pressure you can feel the joints.

When using firmer or deeper pressure, it is important to keep your hand shaped on the body. Grabbing the patient forcefully or quickly will stimulate muscle guarding. You can slowly increase your pressure over a period of time, allowing the patient to make ongoing sensorimotor adjustments to the new information.

Graded pressure combined with movement can have an inhibitory effect on abnormal muscle tone. The movement may vary in its excursion, but the direction is linear rather than circular. Think about moving through the barrier rather than around it. NEVER FORCE your way through the spasticity. Move the body part to the end of the existing range. Maintain your pressure at the place where the movement is restricted. Wait until you feel the restriction soften and the range in movement increase. Follow the increase in range to the next area of restriction. Wait again for a softening of the spasticity. You can add small excursions of movement at the end range to dissipate the restriction.

Deep pressure will give you a different level of proprioceptive information. With deep pressure you receive and send information into the muscles, bones, and joints. When you add deep pressure to graded movement, patients feel the sensation of balanced muscle coactivation around a joint. They can respond above and below the contact point of your hands. As you gradually lighten your pressure, you give them their control back. Your lighter touch feels and follows their movements. Treatment resembles a rather graceful dance, with both partners sharing the lead. We lead, they respond; they lead, we respond.

INTERMITTENT TOUCH

Intermittent touch can be used with patients who potentially have the movement available to them but cannot yet combine the components functionally. Your fingertips or whole hand lightly touch the patient, with your contact on and then off. Your intermittent touch guides them, but the patient does not rely on it being there. The focus is on facilitation rather than inhibition. This can benefit patients who are close to establishing reliable postural reactions or those who can perform a functional skill with some motor cues.

Treatment with Movement—Slow Movement

Combining touch and movement keeps the patient dynamically active. By "movement" I mean a change in the patient's center of gravity (a weight shift), active reach, random movement, or involvement in a specific functional task.

The therapist can lead the movement, follow the patient's movement, or intermittently lead and intermittently follow. Slow movement with a light touch encourages maximum control on the part of the patient. Feel your own body work as you move in slow motion. Sustained coactivation around the joints is required for slow movement (Figure 6). Children with spastic diplegia have a tendency to move very quickly, lunging from one position to another. They use their own momentum and gravity to take them through a transition. In gait, they fall from one foot to the other. When you slow their movements, they initially lose control and collapse into your arms. They may need slow movement to help them improve their control in space.

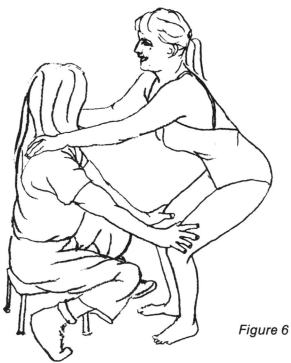

Figure 6

FAST MOVEMENT

Increasing the speed of your facilitation can encourage balance reactions and protective responses. Swift movements can guide you and your patient through a transitional movement pattern that the patient would normally resist. Vary your speed according to the response of the patient and your functional goal.

Treatment with Compression and Traction

As we use touch and movement in our gravity-bound environment, we send messages to the musculoskeletal system. In fact, gravity is sending similar messages to the body in the form of compression and traction. When we stand upright, the weight-bearing joints, from the soles of the feet to the tip of the head, are compressed or pushed closer together. The non-weight-bearing limbs are tractioned by the force of gravity pulling the arm toward the ground. When any force is strong enough to create a separation in the surfaces of the joint, we refer to it as distraction. How strong is the force of gravity on the dangling arms? It is strong enough that most people look for a place to put their hands, a place to plug in some compression. We often stand with a hand lightly weight-bearing into a pocket, on a hip, against a wall, leaning on a table, or hands clasped together in midline. When your arms are tractioned by gravity, the muscles respond by becoming concentrically active around the joints. Over a long period of time your arms fatigue, and you search for mild compression and a warm place to rest.

In standing, the weight-bearing joints are significantly compressed. For example, people waiting in a long line can be seen shifting from one foot to another. Static weight-bearing is exhausting. People who are frequent air travelers know the fatigue of sitting in one small spot. Like everything else, the body thrives on balance—balance between stability and mobility, compression and traction.

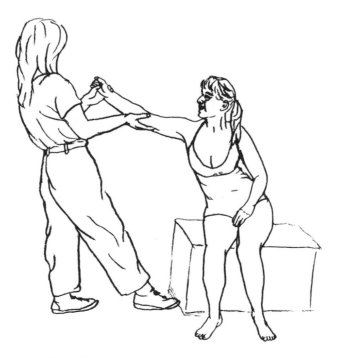

Figure 7

As our hands interact with the movements of our patients, we naturally contribute to compression and traction, sending important information to the musculoskeletal system. We may guide the patient's weight shift with a gentle slow pull on an arm (Figure 7), waiting for the rest of the body to follow and take over the movement. We can compress unilaterally through the rib cage to facilitate the same response (Figure 8).

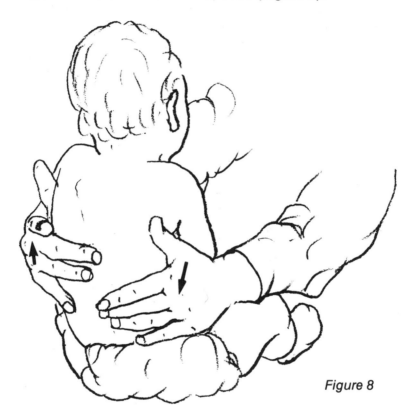

Figure 8

SUSTAINED JOINT TRACTION

Slow sustained traction can release restricted fascia and elongate short musculature, reducing the intensity of hypertonicity, allowing for greater range of movement. Sustained traction is not used forcefully. I take up the slack of the restricted area, maintain the traction, and wait for an increase in movement range. When it comes, I again take up the slack and wait for a further release of the restriction. This is a helpful technique when the patient has a narrow, tight upper chest (Figure 9) and a highly positioned rib cage with or without rib flaring (Figure 10). Use of sustained joint traction in neurodevelopmental treatment can be integrated with concepts of myofascial release (Upledger and Vredevoogd 1983).

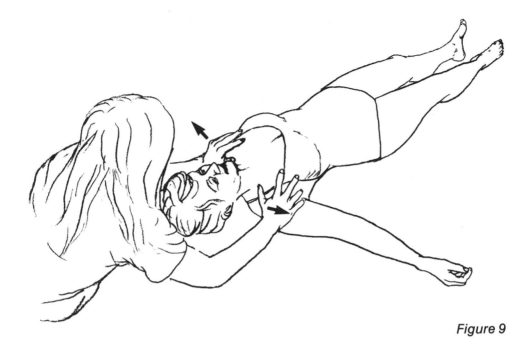

Figure 9

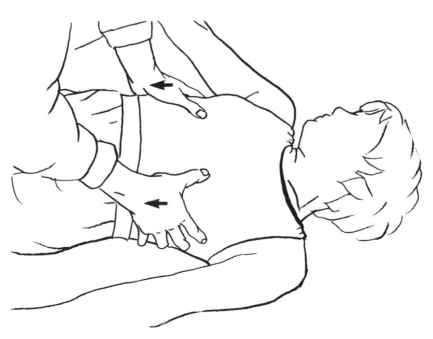

Figure 10

SUSTAINED JOINT COMPRESSION

Sustained light joint compression can be used to facilitate holding, which is the ability to sustain a position. For example, joint compression through the top of the head, toward the pelvis, will help facilitate head and oculomotor control, sending important sensory information through the spine and into the weight-bearing surface (Figure 11). Light joint compression is barely felt by the patient; it is little more than the weight of your hands. This input has a tendency to calm and center the patient, so it is a useful technique for the patient with fluctuating muscle tone, sensory disorganization, and central nervous system irritability. Increasing joint compression is appropriate only when it is directed into properly aligned weight-bearing joints.

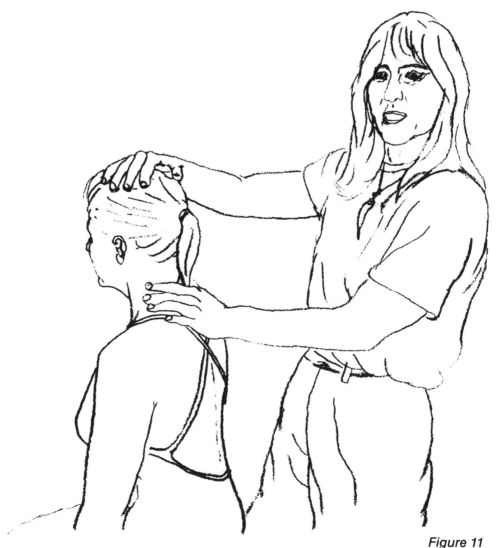

Figure 11

INTERMITTENT COMPRESSION

Repetitive intermittent compression into well-aligned joints can facilitate co-activation around the joints, giving a patient the stimulus needed to maintain posture upright against gravity. The therapist's hands are placed above the joints to be compressed and each stimulus is followed by another. The hands remain in contact with the patient's body throughout the input. The hands create a brief force toward the weight-bearing surface and release the force without removing the hands (Figure 12). Each input builds upon the other until sustained tone gradually develops. When you feel the patient holding the posture under your hands, you can ease up on your intermittent support and let the patient experience self-control of posture. This approach is often referred to as approximation or pressure tapping.

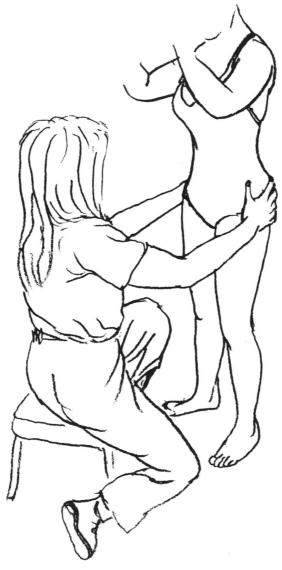

Figure 12

Approximation can be used to facilitate holding and placing in the patient with fluctuating muscle tone. It can be very effective in baby treatment, especially when combined with small ranges of movement (Figure 13). It sets the program for early head and trunk control.

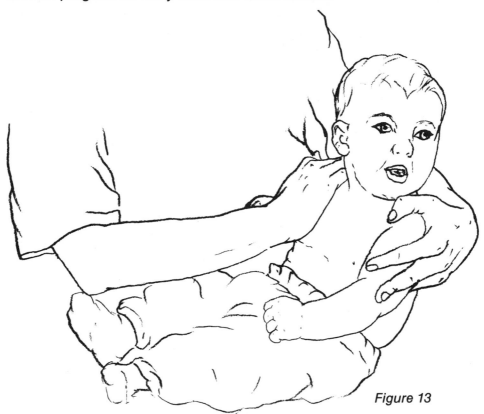

Figure 13

OTHER FORMS OF TAPPING

Tapping is another intermittent sensory input. It is directed at the muscles themselves. Tapping is used when there is apparent or real weakness of specific muscle groups or general hypotonia. It is not used with hypertonicity. Tapping produces an increase in tone and contractibility of muscles due to recruitment of central nervous system impulses. It often takes a series of taps before a response can be noticed. Each tap should be followed quickly by another. It is the repetition that builds up the tone and enables the patient to hold the activity. The therapist's hand does break contact with the patient's body between each tap. Keeping your hand shaped like the body part will allow the input to feel like a gentle clap rather than a slap (Figure 14). Tapping can be used dynamically by creating a "sweep" as you make contact with the body. The "tap" activates the muscles while the "sweep" facilitates a movement by therapeutically altering the alignment (Figure 15).

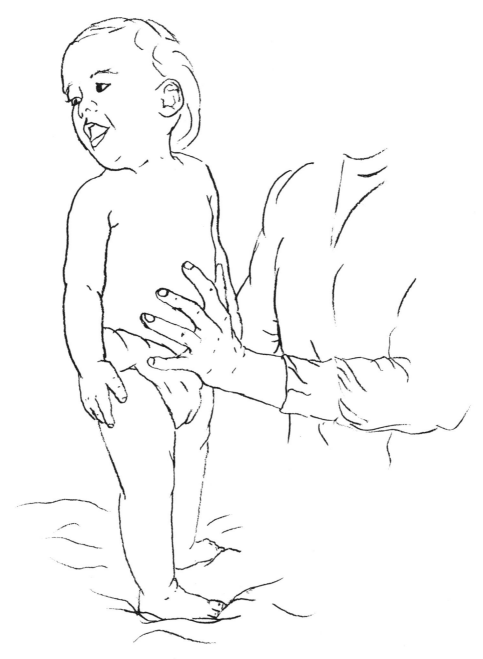

Figure 14

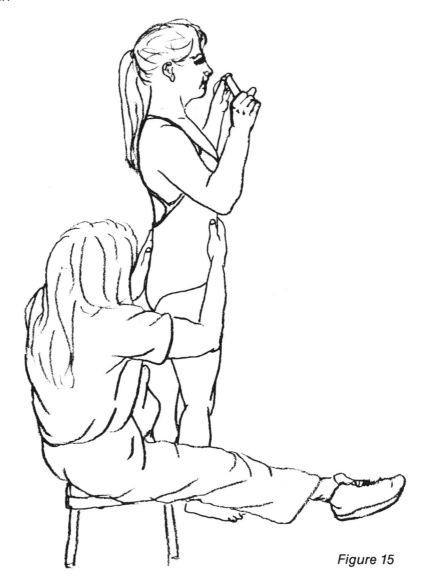

Figure 15

THE CONCEPT OF ASSESSMENT

The first thing I do when a patient comes in for therapy is observe unassisted movements. When the patient is wheelchair-bound, I watch the person function from the chair. If the patient is young, I watch the child function in the caretaker's lap or I observe as the child plays on the floor. Which goal-directed activities can be done independently and efficiently? Which activities are able to be accomplished with dysfunctional control? Which activities can be performed with my assistance? The information gathered from these observations provides long-term direction to the treatment program.

I also spend time talking to the patient. What activities are important to the patient? What are the long-term goals? When the patient is a young child, I investigate the concerns of the caretakers. Are my long-term goals compatible with the goals of the patient? For example, parents often express a strong desire for their child to walk; I may feel it critical that the child develop use of the arms and hands for self-care. Can the acquisition of my long-term goals support the goals of the caretaker or patient?

THE CONCEPT OF CARRYOVER

When the focus of treatment coincides with the patient's needs, we are more likely to achieve carryover of the desired movements outside of treatment. This carryover is essential because dysfunctional movement patterns are habituated. New patterns must be used repeatedly outside of therapy before they too can become habituated. The hope is that the new movement "program" will eventually override the old.

THE CONCEPT OF TREATMENT

New patterns of movement are established in treatment by filling in the missing pieces or component parts of a desired movement. This implies that we will analyze the component parts of the task along with the component parts of the patient's current movement patterns as the task is attempted. What is preventing the patient's success at a specific task? What part of the movement is counterproductive? How can I inhibit the problem? What part of the movement is missing? How can I facilitate that missing component?

We seem to have a great need to get the patient looking good, very quickly. It is most beneficial to take our time and enjoy our interactions with the patient. I work for small, sustained changes that build on one another until collectively they express a coordinated, purposeful, and reliable functional skill.

The treatment techniques described in this chapter will alter the sensorimotor repertoire of your patients. But the ultimate goal of treatment is functional independence. Your treatment techniques, then, will be integrated into functional skills that the patient uses without the assistance of your hands. I spend a brief period of time at the beginning and end of each treatment session assessing the patient's current level of function. I ask myself: Did today's treatment improve the functional independence of this patient? Did I make a difference?

In subsequent chapters, we will deal with the analysis and development of functional movement—common problems found in our patients—along with specific treatment techniques. The material will have a specialized focus on upper extremity function.

References

Bobath, K. 1980. *A neurophysiological basis for the treatment of cerebral palsy.* London: William Heinemann Medical Books Ltd.

Upledger, J., and J. Vredevoogd. 1983. *Craniosacral therapy.* Seattle, WA: Eastland Press.

CHAPTER 2

The Role of the Shoulder Girdle in Posture and Movement

Prologue

A family brought their six-month-old baby to my clinic for a consultation. The referring therapist was also present and described the baby's progress in therapy along with the current problem. During the development of symmetry, the child had established a habit of holding the left hand against the left cheek. The therapist was concerned that the unusual posturing would interfere with the child's use of symmetrical movement. She was also concerned that the left shoulder and elbow might be exhibiting early tonus problems.

As I slowly inhibited the hand-to-cheek posturing, the child became agitated. She not only wanted her hand on her cheek, but she needed it there for postural security. During the first half of the treatment session, I gradually encouraged her to give up this posture. Initially her breathing became disorganized, her eyes drifted in opposite directions, her tongue pulled into retraction, and the head and neck followed the tongue by extending. I reduced her agitation and stabilized her respiratory and oral motor responses by providing deep symmetrical pressure through the rib cage.

When the child was calm, I gradually removed my hands and a full-blown asymmetric reaction reared its ugly head. I had eliminated a compensatory or adaptive pattern and exposed the major problem. The child had not developed symmetry at all. She had found a way to stay in the middle, but had sacrificed one arm to accomplish this midline posture. I felt a moment of panic because the problem I had exposed looked much worse than the adapted pattern she had been using.

The focus of the last half of treatment was the facilitation of symmetrical flexion and extension within very small ranges and in all positions. I wanted to offer the patient components of movement that could replace the asymmetry that forced her to adapt. I offered her a dynamically stable trunk with freer movements of all extremities. I consistently visualized my hands building in symmetry. The child looked better when she left the clinic.

The end result for this patient may have been the use of one arm for postural stability and the other arm for function. In time, she would find other adaptations as she was encouraged to move in and out of positions, reach with both arms, feed herself, communicate, and play. All of her adaptations would be some variation of asymmetrical fixation.

Without symmetry, the extremities compromise function in order to help the head and trunk establish a relationship with gravity. Consequently, we must approach upper extremity treatment from a whole-body perspective.

The Value of Symmetry

Officially, the shoulder girdle is comprised of the humerus, scapula, clavicle, and sternum. However, considering the extensive kinesiology involved and the relationship of shoulder girdle movement to general body motion, I include the rib cage, spine, head, and pelvis as essential parts of dynamic shoulder girdle control. The pieces of the shoulder complex move rhythmically or in synchrony with each other and with the whole body.

In order to neutralize gravity, a balance between symmetrical flexion and extension is necessary. This unique position is the body's frame of reference for all movements. Efficient movement works off this central axis. Managing midline allows us to control posture and movement, while we use the extremities for functions such as dressing, feeding, and protective extension. If this balance is impossible to achieve, the patient must use the extremities to help control posture. This, of course, is at the expense of function and safety. Symmetry, then, is an appropriate place to begin our study of the shoulder girdle.

Symmetrical Control of Posture

When there is a change in the center of gravity, the shoulder girdle moves or glides on the rib cage in response to movement of the spine. For example, as the body moves behind the center of gravity, the shoulders move forward and up, contributing to a symmetrical flexion response as the body rights itself against gravity (Figure 16). The arms can follow the shoulders by moving forward as well (Figure 17). The spine lengthens the back, and the head flexes on the neck. The abdominals contract to flex or shorten the torso in front. If the weight shift is significant, the abdominals tilt the top of the pelvis posteriorly, behind the hips. This dynamic flexion response prevents a backward fall by moving the body forward. Throughout this automatic postural reaction, the extensors are working eccentrically, or in a lengthened position, to prevent a response of excessive flexion. As the body nears the center of gravity, the extensors work concentrically or in a shortened position to straighten the spine.

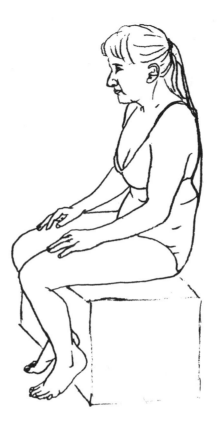

Figure 16

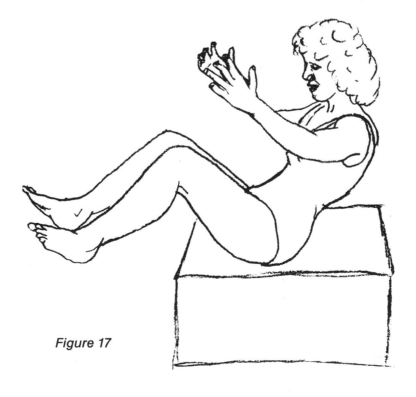

Figure 17

On the other hand, symmetrical extension prevents us from falling on our face when the body moves in front of the center of gravity. With this forward movement, the spine extends or shortens in the back and the head extends on the spine. The shoulders move back with a visible broadening of the upper chest (Figure 18). The arms can follow with movement back toward

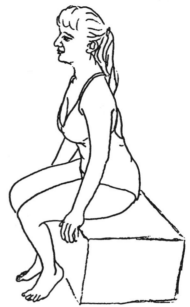

Figure 18

abduction or extension (Figure 19). If the weight shift is significant, the top of the pelvis moves forward, in front of the hips. The front of the torso becomes longer. Throughout this postural reaction, the trunk flexors work eccentrically to prevent a response of excessive extension. As the body returns to the middle, flexors and extensors work together or co-contract to maintain this efficient relationship with gravity, freeing the extremities for function.

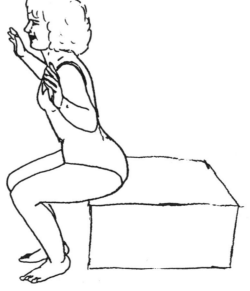

Figure 19

When symmetrical control is not available, the patient will search for and use postural adaptations. The patient with hemiparesis illustrates this adaptive process. Because both shoulders are not equally active, the patient will use an excessive forward movement in one shoulder while the other shoulder lags markedly behind (Figure 20). In other words, the

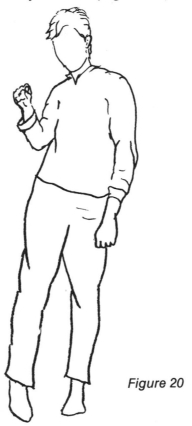

Figure 20

patient will overreact on one side of the body to compensate for the inactivity on the other side of the body. In order to make this adaptation more efficient, the patient can fixate or strongly posture the arm connected to the inactive shoulder. This reduces the sensation of "dragging" the shoulder along during movement. This fixation will intensify as the patient attempts to increase speed.

The same adaptation is repeated in the trunk and pelvis: one side is overactive and the other is dragged along with the movement. The inactive side of the trunk is held in a shortened position with the pelvis hiked and often anteriorly rotated. This asymmetrical elevation in the pelvis creates a functional leg length discrepancy. Consequently, during ambulation, the patient develops plantar flexion to equalize the leg lengths.

Although this description describes specific problems related to hemiparesis, the adaptation is evident at all levels of central nervous system involvement where symmetry never developed or was lost as a result of injury.

Unilateral Control of Posture

With a lateral weight shift, the spine lengthens on the weight-bearing side and shortens on the side that is unweighted (Figure 21). The torso uses concentric unilateral flexion and extension to shorten the unweighted side. Eccentric unilateral flexion and extension allow active lengthening on the weighted side. Each side's respective flexors and extensors have a specific job in controlling this weight shift, righting the head and body in space, and bringing the person back to the middle.

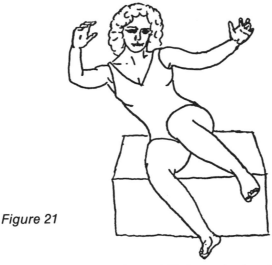

Figure 21

Many patients attempt to weight shift laterally by dropping the shoulder toward the weight-bearing surface (Figure 22). They flex into gravity. They shift their weight through the upper body rather than through the pelvis and hips. This inability to control the lateral weight shift will interfere with independent dressing (particularly lower body dressing), hygiene, extended reach, and ambulation. In actuality, this adapted pattern interferes with weight shifting in all positions.

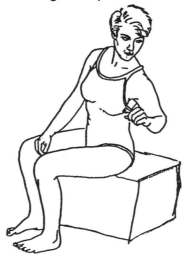

Figure 22

Diagonal Control

When a lateral weight shift propels the individual too far for straight-plane lateral control to prevent a fall, diagonal postural reactions are needed. This means that the upper body can rotate over the hips and pelvis (Figure 23).

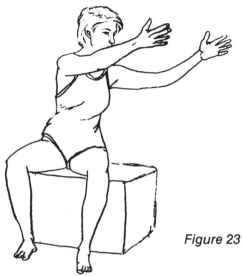

Figure 23

There are two different ways to respond with rotation. An individual can rotate with extension where the upper body and expanded shoulders turn toward the weight-bearing hip (Figure 24). Conversely, the individual can

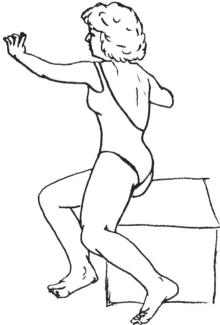

Figure 24

rotate with flexion, where the upper body with protracted shoulders turns away from the weight-bearing hip (Figure 25). In both cases, the opposite shoulder and pelvis orient toward each other. Rotation with extension develops before rotation with flexion. The use of diagonal patterns relies on the development of straight plane control.

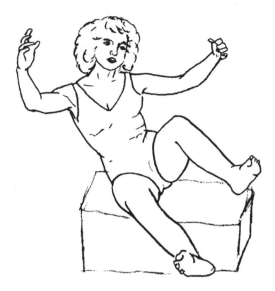

Figure 25

Dynamic Sitting

The ability to weight shift and return to the center is necessary in all positions. However, in terms of self-care independence, performance in school, and economic freedom, we are specifically concerned with upper body control from a dynamic sitting base. Consequently, upper extremity treatment includes strategies that impact on the trunk and hip control needed for sitting. Appendix C will broaden and clarify your knowledge base of the spine, pelvis, and hips as they relate to sitting.

In Chapter 3, we begin our focus on upper extremity treatment from a whole-body perspective. Take this journey slowly and allow yourself adequate time to integrate and apply the material to your clinical practice.

CHAPTER 3

Analysis and Treatment for Horizontal Reach

When the shoulder girdle is working in synchrony with the torso, the upper arm has the potential for quality function. The shoulder girdle makes it possible for the upper arm to project the hand in a wide range of space. The shoulder girdle makes it possible for the humerus to maintain or hold its position in space as we brush our teeth or indulge in that delicious pizza. The shoulders make it possible for the humerus to follow a moving target. This means that the arm can change directions in mid movement.

When the shoulder girdle is working in synchrony with the torso, the humerus can accept partial body weight and move it around. In other words, the humerus can be stable on a surface and support the torso as it moves over and around the weight-bearing arm.

When assessing the shoulder girdle, then, observe what the upper arm is doing during reach and weight bearing. The quality of humeral control shows us how well the shoulder parts are working together. This chapter will investigate the shoulder through upper arm function in a horizontal plane. It will focus on treatment techniques based on an understanding of the process of normal development. Understanding development is important to therapists working with adults, as well as with children, since the analysis provides critical information about how components of movement emerge through successive approximation. Treatment intervention strives to plug in those same movement components for function in a way that the central nervous system can understand and use them.

Movements of the Arm in a Horizontal Plane

HORIZONTAL HUMERAL ABDUCTION

Analysis of component parts

Movement of the humerus toward horizontal abduction or in a ninety-degree range is coupled with (1) scapular adduction or movement of the scapula toward the spine, (2) thoracic extension, and (3) a posterior movement of the clavicle in its horizontal plane (Kapandji 1982). This pattern of movement is used by developing children to reinforce antigravity extension as new postures evolve. The movement is also used during wide-range reach, when lengthening an object such as a water hose, or spreading an item like a bed sheet. Humeral abduction is critical when we use an arm to push ourselves out of sidelying, to get off the floor or out of bed.

The middle deltoid and supraspinatus abduct the humerus ninety degrees without the help of the shoulder girdle (Figure 26). The middle trapezius adducts the scapula with the help of the rhomboids (Figure 27). Spinal extensors straighten the thoracic spine enough to allow the clavicle to move backward and expand the chest.

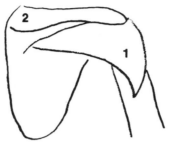

Figure 26

1. Middle deltoid
2. Supraspinatus

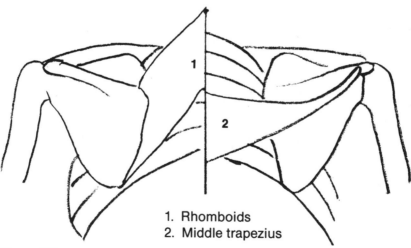

1. Rhomboids
2. Middle trapezius

Figure 27

Analysis of development

The full-term infant exhibits an initial posture of physiological flexion due primarily to the position of the fetus in utero. The shoulders are elevated and the scapulae are abducted (Figure 28). The arms are adducted and flexed. This physiological flexion keeps the infant "collected" or held together through the transition from the compact uterus to our spacious, gravity-bound environment. This early flexion is a point of stability for infant movement, meaning it stabilizes muscle origins so that the child can randomly move the body.

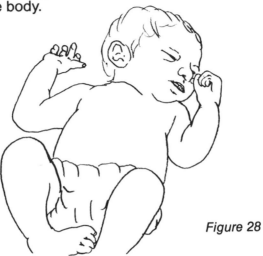

Figure 28

The behavior of the premature infant provides an example of new life without physiological flexion (Figure 29). These infants may vacillate between irritability and passive motor behavior. Initially they cannot find a way to feel posturally secure and do not have the mechanical stability to initiate early random movement of their bodies. Moreover, this inability interferes with breathing and the oral control needed for food intake.

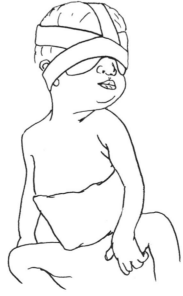

Figure 29

A number of factors contribute to the full-term infant's ability to progress from a snugly compact posture to one where the shoulders are broad, the spine is straight, and the arms move freely away from the rib cage. When the infant is in supine, the spine is held in extension against the supporting surface. The scapula is maintained next to the ribs. The force of gravity on the anterior portion of the body encourages the shoulders to move back against the supporting surface (Figure 30). The frequent random movements generate humeral movements away from the body toward horizontal abduction. The infant is not using voluntary isolated humeral muscles. The momentum for random movement is generated throughout the body. Initially this movement of extremities in space is frightening for the infant. The parent can respond to subsequent crying by swaddling or holding the child with the extremities close to the body. But within a short period of time the infant begins to enjoy the sensation of random movement and by twelve weeks of age will try to duplicate interesting movement sensations.

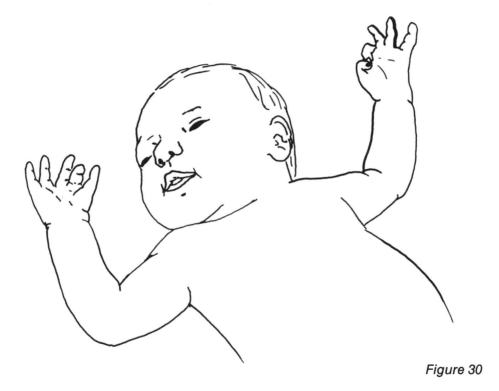

Figure 30

By two months of age, physiological flexion has decreased and the infant feels somewhat floppy or hypotonic. However, the infant continues to engage in random movements by working off the stability provided by the

ATNR or asymmetrical posturing (Figure 31). This fencing posture is off midline with the exception of bilateral humeral abduction. The shoulders then become an important focal point for development. This is active humeral abduction at a ninety-degree plane with enough scapular and spinal activity to support head turning with eye tracking. It also supports the early asymmetrical swiping movement of the arm in addition to generalized body motion. Because the stability is located in the shoulders, the greatest range of random movement is expressed above and below the shoulders. What we see is an increase in the range and control of head movement as well as an increase in range of spine and pelvic movement (Figure 32). The shoulder girdle and arms act as one working unit and create the image of being "wind swept." As one shoulder elevates, the other shoulder depresses. A straight line can be drawn between one humeral head and the other.

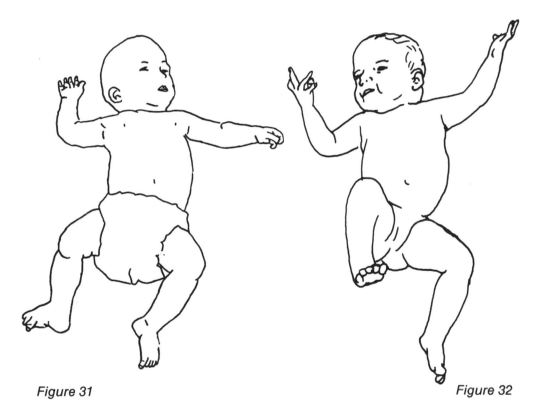

Figure 31   *Figure 32*

In addition, the shoulders and arms are used for early antigravity control of posture. The child uses active horizontal abduction of the arms in the landau at five months (Figure 33), to reinforce sitting at six months (Figure 34), and to reinforce standing at the end of the first year of life (Figure 35). As the arms abduct, the scapula moves close to the spine, biomechanically reinforcing spinal extension. The shoulders help straighten and keep the spine straight. As endurance and strength of isolated spinal extensors improve, the arms are free to move forward for function.

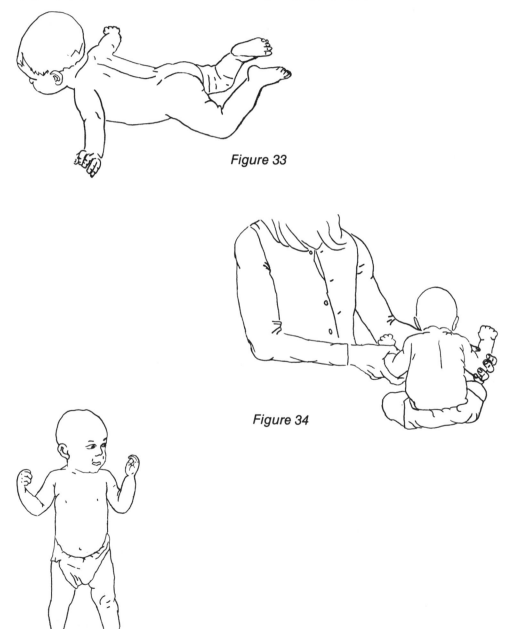

Figure 33

Figure 34

Figure 35

Active horizontal abduction of the arm is used for transitional movement patterns. From sidelying, the child pushes the arm against the surface using humeral abduction (Figure 36). Because the surface prevents isolated movement of the humerus, the torso is lifted. The child can then stop the movement in sidelying forearm prop or can continue the movement until the child lands on the tummy. From the side prop position, the child will eventually lean forward, transferring the body weight from the forearm to the hand, using elbow extension to raise the body up into side prop (Figure 37).

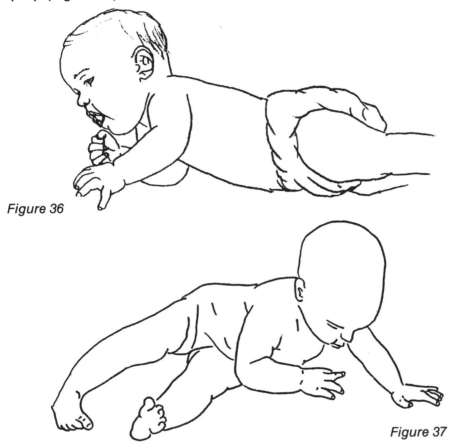

Figure 36

Figure 37

Assessment and treatment to improve function

Spasticity, shortened musculature, and subsequent tissue restriction in the upper chest will prevent the patient from broadening the shoulders. This in turn interferes with humeral abduction and thoracic extension. A strong pull from the pectorals, for example, will hold the scapula in an elevated, abducted, and anteriorly tipped position (Figure 38). This will limit upper respiratory function by restricting rib cage expansion during inhalation (Figure 39). A strong pull into protraction and elevation with thoracic flexion will interfere with the development of head control and cause a compensatory pattern of head and neck hyperextension (Figure 40). The head and neck will overextend to compensate for the lack of extension in the thoracic spine.

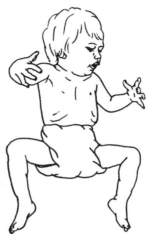

Figure 38

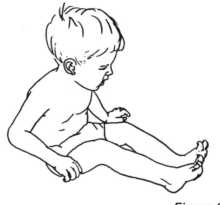

Figure 39

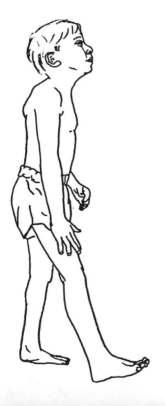

Figure 40

Releasing upper chest tightness can be accomplished unilaterally by gently stabilizing the sternum while slowly moving the shoulder toward the weight-bearing surface (Figure 41). You also can move the shoulders, bilaterally, toward the weight-bearing surface (Figure 42). Move the shoulders to the end of the available range, hold it there and wait for a reduction in the spasticity. As the tone softens, you follow the expansion to the next available range and hold it there. Wait for the next reduction in tone and again follow the increase in range of movement. You can repeat this cycle until the level of spasticity stops changing or full expansion is achieved. It is best to facilitate ample active movement once you have inhibited the abnormal muscle tone. With the exception of severely spastic patients, the focus is on facilitation. Pushing the shoulders through the tone rapidly will not reduce the spasticity. Techniques used when the patient is in supine are beneficial since thoracic extension is supported by the weight-bearing surface and the scapula is supported against the ribs.

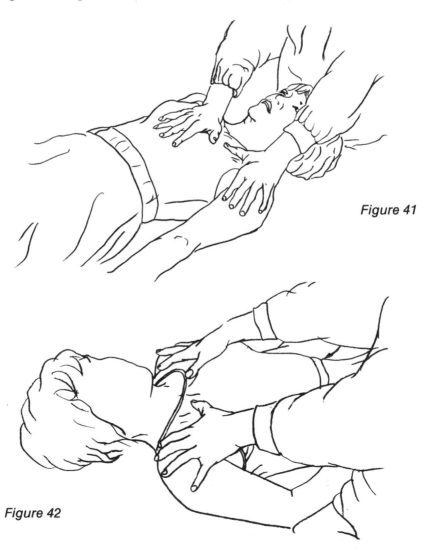

Figure 41

Figure 42

However, the supine position tends to be a passive place to work with patients. Consequently, as you feel a decrease in the upper chest tightness, encourage your patient to reach toward the side, move the head and neck, breathe deeply, or vocalize. This treatment approach may be utilized with the patient in a sitting position by moving the patient against the therapist (Figure 43) or against the seat back of a chair.

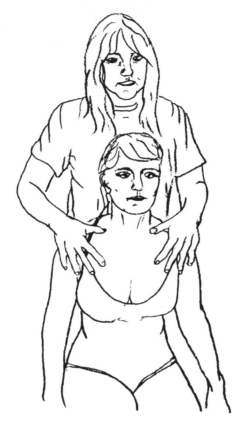

Figure 43

Problems involving restricted passive movement between the head, neck, and shoulder girdle may be treated prior to facilitation techniques. Sustained light traction on the occiput or base of the skull will reduce tightness between the head and the neck (Figure 44). Stabilizing the

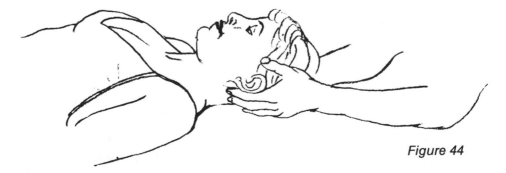

Figure 44

occiput with one hand and moving the shoulder away from it will release the shoulder from head and neck (Figure 45). Remember to work slowly, never forcing against the spasticity. As you feel a softening of the restriction and an increase in range of lateral head and neck movement, slowly rotate the head to increase the elongation (Figure 46). You may then

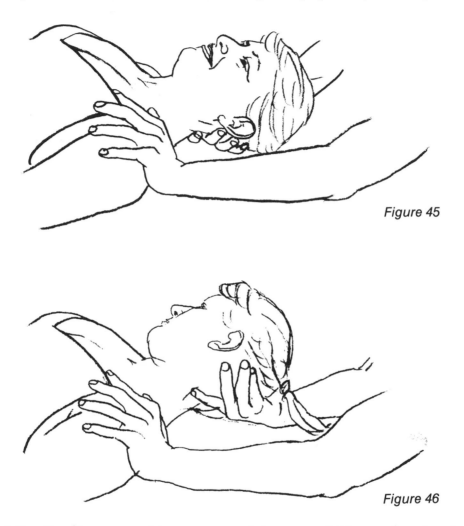

Figure 45

Figure 46

stabilize the rib cage and encourage maintenance of this new freedom in movement as the patient turns the head to look around, inhales with freer movement of the shoulders, and reaches. Light traction applied to the sacrum in a caudal direction will lengthen the cervical spine (Figure 47). This technique reduces extensor spasticity along the length of the whole spine, reducing tightness between the pelvis and spine as well.

When spasticity prevents the upper arm from moving freely away from the rib cage, treatment will be directed to the area of the axilla. Stabilize the upper rib cage and gently move the upper arm away from the ribs (Figure 48). The longer you maintain this elongation, the less the rebound. You can also stabilize the humerus as you gently move the upper ribs away from

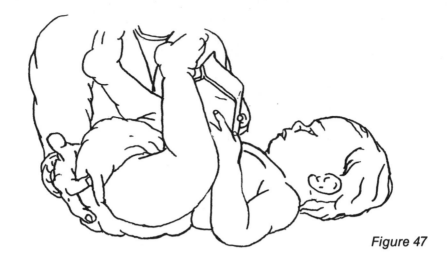

Figure 47

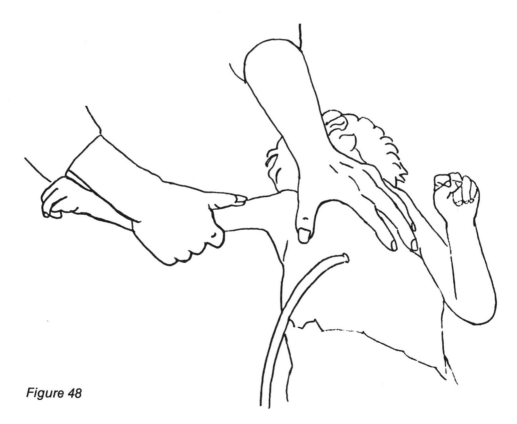

Figure 48

the arm (Figure 49). As your hand shapes itself on your patient's ribs, lightly compress or push in while you gently move the ribs in the direction of the feet.

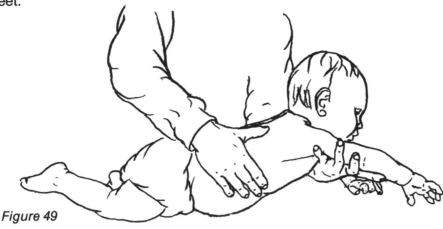

Figure 49

Lack of active scapular adduction and thoracic spinal extension can prolong the patient's need to use humeral abduction to support spinal extension. In this situation, you can facilitate the desired activity by supporting the humerus, elbows, or wrist. The elbows may be flexed or extended, as long as neutral rotation of the humerus is maintained. In prone, abduct the patient's upper arms (Figure 50). Outward bilateral traction (a gentle force) will prevent shoulder protraction. Lift the patient's upper chest off of the weight-bearing surface and wait for a response to your facilitation by actively lifting the head, adducting the scapulae and

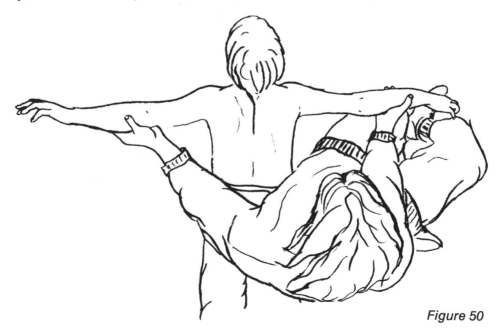

Figure 50

extending the spine between the scapulae. The patient's motor response should be initiated in the head and neck and not the low back or hips. When you use this treatment approach in sitting (Figure 51) and standing (Figure 52), remember to keep your patient's upper body in front of the center of

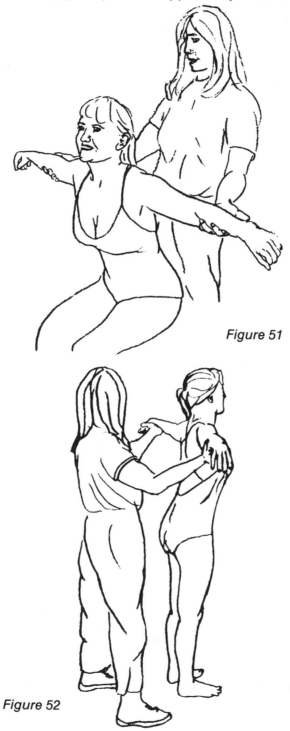

Figure 51

Figure 52

gravity where extension is an appropriate postural response. This may also be accomplished in side prop (Figure 53). Once the patient responds, encourage holding of the posture to increase strength and endurance. Over time, your patient will be able to maintain an erect spine while the arms are free for function.

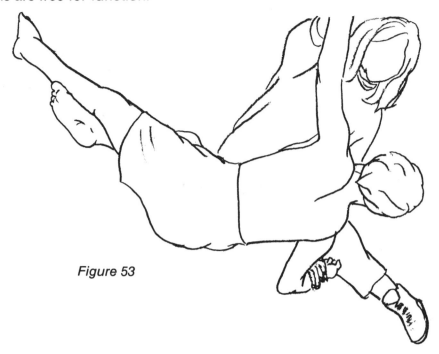

Figure 53

Immobility of the thoracic spine can be reduced by several general techniques. You can apply gentle downward and inward pressure to the ribs as the patient moves or has help moving the arms (Figure 54). The

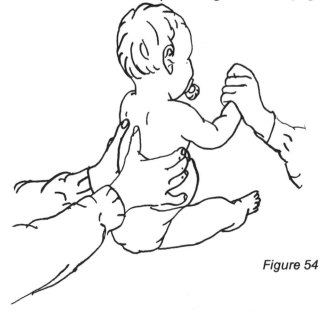

Figure 54

patient can be positioned supine over a large therapy ball. The patient is gently bounced on the ball while the therapist expands the width of the upper chest (Figure 55). The use of inversion will facilitate spinal extension, and gravity will help release the arm from the trunk (Figure 56). A larger

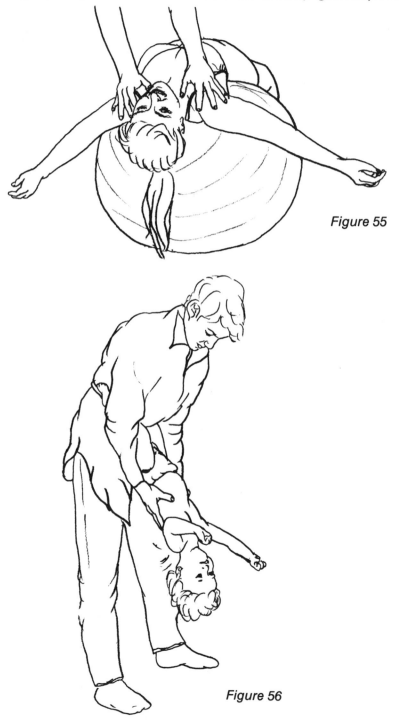

Figure 55

Figure 56

patient can be partially inverted over a ball (Figure 57). Allow gravity to expand the chest as you stabilize the torso. In sitting you can lift the patient's upper chest while you stabilize the spine or pelvis (Figure 58).

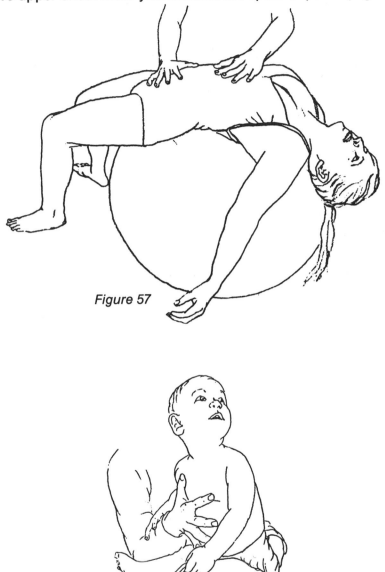

Figure 57

Figure 58

HORIZONTAL HUMERAL ADDUCTION

Analysis of component parts

Movement of the humerus toward horizontal humeral adduction/flexion or movement of the humerus toward midline at a 90-degree plane is coupled with (1) scapular abduction, or movement of the scapula away from the spine, (2) thoracic flexion, and (3) an anterior movement of the clavicle in its horizontal plane. This is an important movement pattern because it brings our two hands together for bilateral tasks. It is important to remember that pure adduction is a movement of the arm toward the ribs, adduction/flexion moves the arm toward midline in front of the ribs, adduction/extension moves the arm behind the ribs.

The anterior deltoid and costo-sternal portion of the pectoralis major adduct and internally rotate the humerus (Figure 59). The serratus anterior and trapezius work together to abduct and stabilize the scapula as it follows the arm (Figure 60). As the scapula abducts, the thoracic spine flexes.

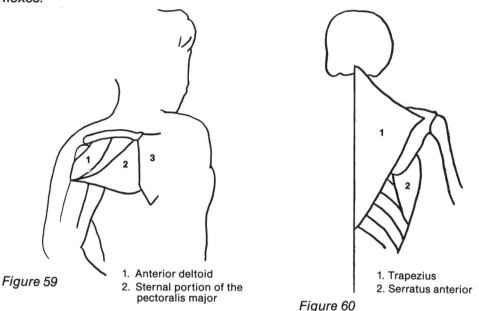

Figure 59

1. Anterior deltoid
2. Sternal portion of the pectoralis major

1. Trapezius
2. Serratus anterior

Figure 60

Analysis of development

The posture of the full-term newborn in prone is one of generalized flexion with the arms positioned in adduction with extension, elbows behind shoulders (Figure 61). Because of the flexion in the spine and hips, the infant bears the majority of body weight on the shoulders, arms, and head. The lower part of the body supports the least amount of weight and is therefore free to move. As the infant randomly moves the legs, additional weight is transferred to the upper body. As the infant lifts and turns the head, an increase in body weight is transferred to the shoulders. Consequently, during movement, the shoulders are bombarded with body weight from two directions. The demand placed on the shoulder girdle in prone stimulates early development of the upper body. The shoulder girdle develops on demand.

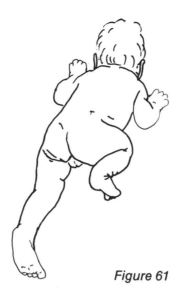

Figure 61

The initial response of the shoulders to the newborn's random movements is to collapse toward the supporting surface. Within a few weeks, however, the shoulders are able to support the weight without a collapse. As physiological flexion decreases, the arms begin to move away from the prone torso. The infant attempts to lift the head and upper chest, but does so asymmetrically (Figure 62).

The three-month-old is able to sustain a more symmetrical head and upper chest lift. The child uses horizontal humeral adduction against the surface, pushing or adducting the arms into the surface. Because the supporting surface prevents isolated arm motion, the upper body is instead lifted up (Figure 63). Because the elbow is now positioned more in line with the shoulder or in front of the ribs, adduction is combined with flexion. Active humeral adduction and abduction are not sufficient to support unweighting of an arm for reach. Consequently, when the three-month-old wants a toy, the child simply lets the shoulders sink to the surface and obtains the toy with the mouth.

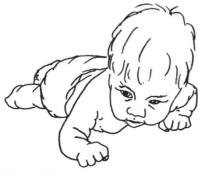

Figure 62

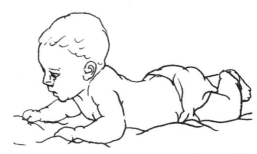

Figure 63

In supine, we see this new humeral motion used functionally. The three-month-old will bring hands toward the midline, using adduction with internal rotation (Figure 64). This movement component is critical for hand-on-body and hand-to-mouth contact. The child uses adduction with neutral rotation for bilateral reaching as well and eventually will use this movement in a wider range for crossing midline.

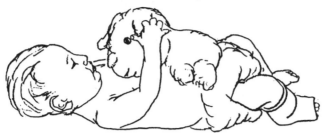

Figure 64

It is important to understand why the young child uses humeral adduction against a surface in prone. Why can the three-month-old reach forward from a supine position when the child has difficulty with the same functional arm pattern in supported sitting? Whenever the arms move in front of the ribs, the scapula moves away from the spine. This mechanically flexes the thoracic spine. In order for the child to maintain trunk control during reach, the lower portion of the spine must extend to balance out the thoracic flexion. Otherwise, each forward movement of the arm would cause a generalized flexor response in the spine. This flexor posturing is a consistent problem for neurologically impaired patients attempting to reach in any position. Since the prone and supine positions support extension of the spine, the developing child learns to use and control isolated humeral movement first with the spine supported by a weight-bearing surface.

Assessing and treating for function
Humeral adduction is at risk when the scapula is unable to abduct on the rib cage or when the clavicle cannot move forward. You can reduce these restrictions by moving your patient's torso over the humerus in sidelying and slightly beyond, toward prone (Figure 65). The same principle of

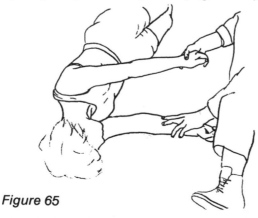

Figure 65

treatment can be applied to the seated patient. By maintaining the arms in a forward position, the patient can lean back or away from you, actively freeing up the shoulder girdle (Figure 66). With one hand maintaining the arms in a forward position and the other hand on the sternum, you can gently move the patient in a posterior direction (Figure 67). You are moving the patient's torso behind the shoulders and arms. As the spine flexes, the shoulders will move forward, liberating the scapula and clavicle. In addition, you have the option of slowly moving the scapulas on the rib cage toward abduction as the patient moves the arms forward (Figure 68).

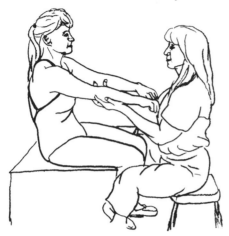

Figure 66

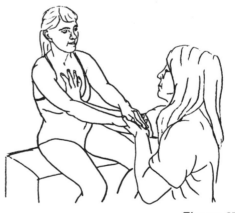

Figure 67

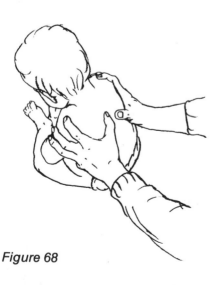

Figure 68

Patients who are unable to combine thoracic flexion with lumbar extension as they attempt to bring their arms in front of the rib cage will be pulled into gravity. As the arms move forward and the shoulders follow with protraction, the thoracic spine will flex, as it should. However, the lumbar spine should not be bound to follow. When it does, it will lead to a generalized flexion response (Figure 69).

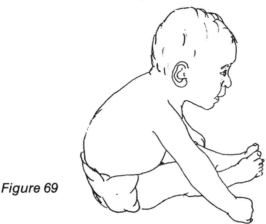

Figure 69

The young patient, in supine, can be encouraged to feel and tolerate upper thoracic flexion with lumbar extension during play. Support the baby's low back and pelvis, allowing gravity to lengthen the anterior portion of the torso. Maintain this position as the baby reaches or plays hand-to-hand (Figure 70).

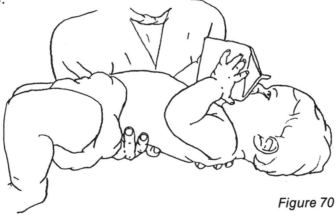

Figure 70

In all patients, the pelvis can be maintained in a slight anterior pelvic tilt during reach (Figure 71). This will provide a stable sitting base for upper body control. Initially you may feel a significant resistance to your attempt to maintain this pelvic tilt, as the patient strives to bring the hands together or close to the body. You can use anterior (Figure 72) or posterior (Figure 73) weight shifting of pelvis over hips to inhibit this spasticity. If you continue to feel resistance, you may be dealing with proximal hamstring tightness rather than restrictions in the low back. The proximal end of the hamstrings can be lengthened by diagonally shifting your patient's pelvis

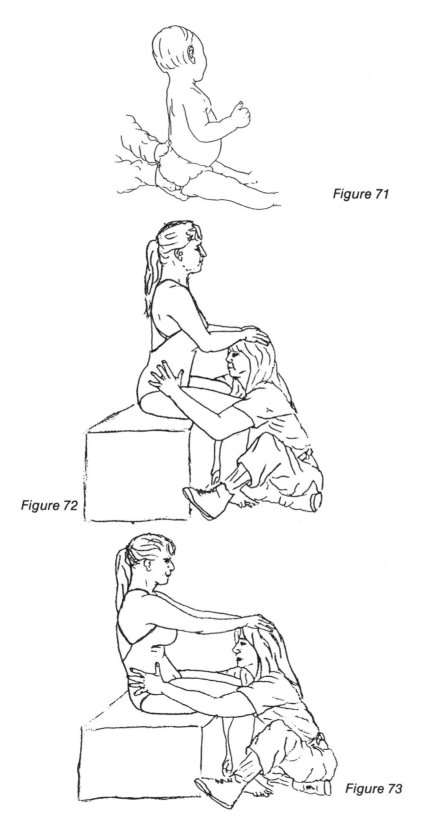

Figure 71

Figure 72

Figure 73

over one hip at a time (Figure 74). Fixed deformities in the low back, pelvis, and hips will prevent the patient from having a stable sitting base.

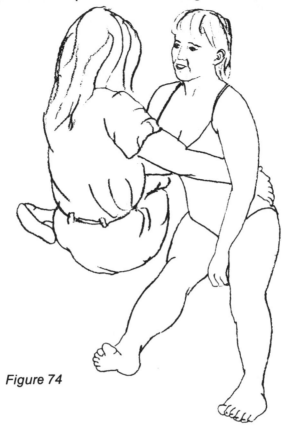

Figure 74

Treatment in prone offers a support that encourages spinal extension and provides a stable surface for abdominal activity. Patients with tight hip flexors will have difficulty shifting their upper body weight to the low abdominal and pelvic region (Figure 75). Inhibition techniques to reduce flexor spasticity or other types of restrictions will help the patient tolerate and enjoy the prone experience. In the normal child, lateral weight shifting in prone lengthens the hip flexors between five and seven months of age.

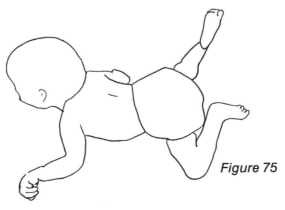

Figure 75

You can shift your patient's weight laterally while you apply gentle sustained pressure through the hip, toward the supporting surface (Figure 76). This will lengthen the flexors, one hip at a time. A gentle traction on the weight-bearing leg, as you use this technique, will encourage further elongation.

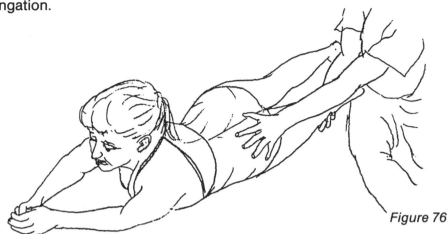

Figure 76

Treatment in prone is not static. Placing a patient in prone prop does not, in and of itself, make the proper demand on the shoulders, because the upper body can virtually "hang" on the ligaments or sink into the weight-bearing arms. The therapeutic use of prone implies that we move the patient in and out of the position with only brief periods of stasis.

To facilitate humeral adduction in prone, you can stabilize the elbows and compress the humerus into the glenoid fossa (Figure 77). Wait for your

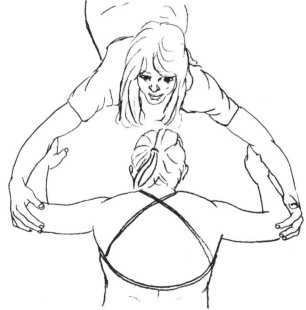

Figure 77

patient to begin the upper chest lift and follow the elbows as they press into the surface (Figure 78). With your help, the elbows will move toward the midline and initially the ribs and spine will sink away from the scapulae (Figure 79). You can expand the width of the shoulders and gently compress the spine to isolate head and neck control and activate the torso

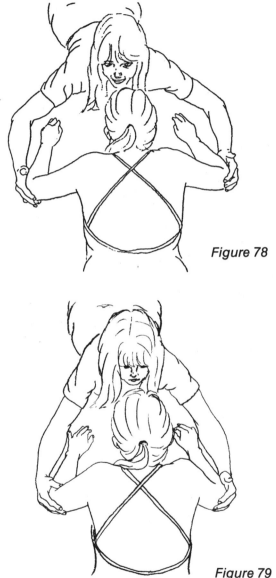

Figure 78

Figure 79

as well (Figure 80). Furthermore, you can compress the rib cage and move it toward the pelvis (Figure 81). This change in your hand placement allows your patient to experience self-control of the shoulder, humerus, head, and neck, working off the stability felt at the rib cage and through the weight-bearing surface. Once prone position can be tolerated, begin to shift the patient's weight from side to side and help the patient to move in and out

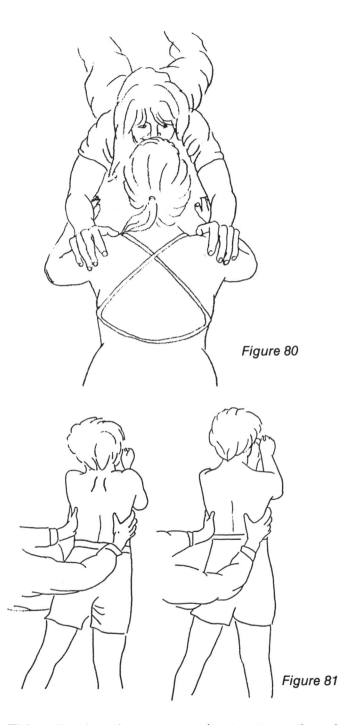

Figure 80

Figure 81

of sidelying. This will give the opportunity to strengthen humeral adduction and abduction which in turn will stimulate improved shoulder girdle control. The shoulders need to be challenged by transitional movements. If your patient is older, work on shifting weight from sidelying to side prop and toward but not fully into prone.

As your patient experiences a decrease in the degree of dysfuctional tonus and an increase in range of movement, you may stimulate active arm movement as a sensorimotor base for function. Consistently include function in your treatment. Facilitation of horizontal humeral movements in reach can be gained through humeral compression (Figure 82), intermittent traction (Figure 83), or external support (Figure 84). This approach encourages holding and placing of the arm. In addition, supporting the gleno-humeral joint (Figure 85), scapula (Figure 86), ribs

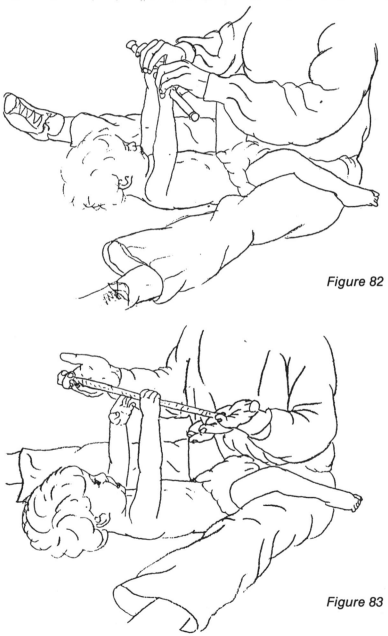

Figure 82

Figure 83

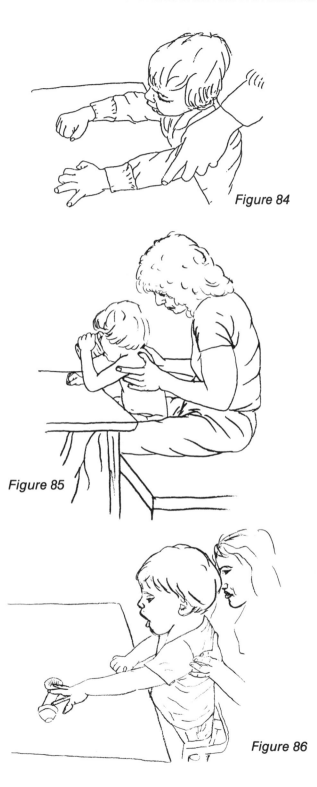

Figure 84

Figure 85

Figure 86

(Figure 87), and low back (Figure 88) will provide adequate stability to increase the range of reach and correct the reach in mid stream.

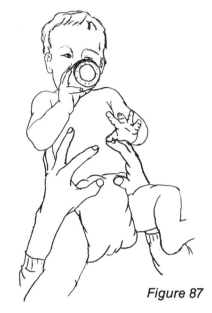

Figure 87

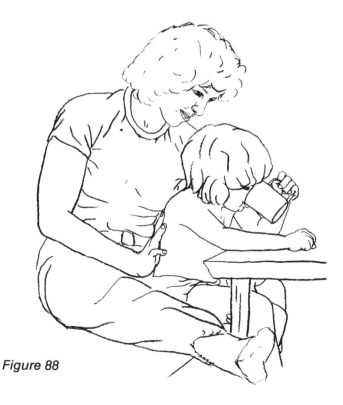

Figure 88

Summary

This is the first part of our journey into arm function. As your patient develops control of the arm within a ninety-degree range, you can prepare for movements above the head and behind the torso. Wide range arm movements require extensive control of the trunk.

References

Kapandji, I. 1982. Upper limb. In *The physiology of the joints,* Vol. I. New York: Churchill Livingstone.

CHAPTER 4

Analysis and Treatment for Wide-Range Reach

As the arm journeys beyond the ninety-degree horizontal plane, it requires an interactive relationship with the spine, ribs, and pelvis. Treatment for wide-range reach therefore will include strategies specifically designed to intervene on problems associated with the torso.

Movements of the Arm Above the Head

HUMERAL FLEXION

Analysis of component parts

Humeral flexion above ninety degrees is coupled with (1) scapular upward rotation or movement of the inferior border of the scapula away from the spine and toward the axilla, (2) thoracic flexion, and (3) upward axial rotation of the clavicle.

The anterior fibers of the deltoid, coraco-brachialis, and clavicular portion of the pectoralis major work together to initiate flexion and project the arm above the head (Figure 89). The shoulder girdle is needed when the arm reaches beyond 60 degrees. The trapezius and seratus anterior rotate the scapula in an upward direction. Even with this cooperative muscle action

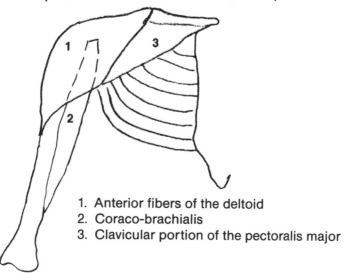

1. Anterior fibers of the deltoid
2. Coraco-brachialis
3. Clavicular portion of the pectoralis major

Figure 89

of the shoulder, complex humeral flexion is limited to 120 degrees, due to the resistance of the latissimus dorsi (Figure 90). In order for the humerus to reach its full potential of 180 degrees, active lumbar extension is needed (Kapandji 1982).

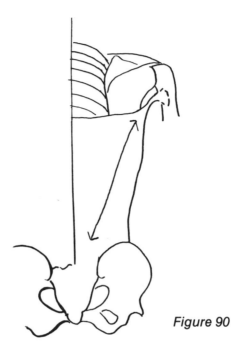

Figure 90

HUMERAL ABDUCTION

Analysis of component parts

Humeral abduction above ninety degrees is coupled with (1) scapular upward rotation or movement of the inferior border of the scapula away from the spine and toward the axilla, (2) thoracic flexion, and (3) upward axial rotation of the clavicle.

The middle fibers of the deltoid and supraspinatus work together to initiate abduction (Figure 91). The shoulder girdle is needed when the arm

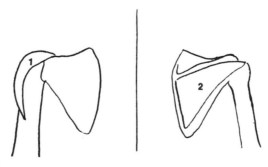

1. Middle deltoid
2. Supraspinatus

Figure 91

reaches beyond ninety degrees. The trapezius and serratus anterior rotate the scapula in an upward direction (Figure 92). Even with this cooperative muscle action of the shoulder, complex humeral abduction is limited to 150 degrees due to the resistance of the latissimus dorsi. In order for the humerus to reach its full potential of 180 degrees, active lumbar extension is required.

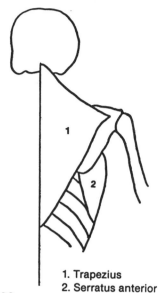

1. Trapezius
2. Serratus anterior

Figure 92

Role of the scapula. Participation of the scapula is essential. Without it, the humerus will not move above the head in either flexion or abduction. The glenoid fossa is small and shallow in relationship to the size of the humeral head (Figure 93). When the scapula is unable to move in synchrony with the humerus, there is inadequate space for the humeral head to move within the bony structure. To further complicate matters, the only bony attachment of the scapula to the body is at the clavicle. When clavicular movements are restricted, the scapular movements become mechanically limited as well.

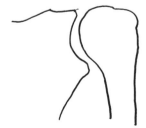

Figure 93

Relationship of serratus anterior to abdominals. In the young child, wide-range humeral flexion and abduction develop in association with capitol (head) flexion on an elongated neck (Figure 94). Humeral flexion also develops in conjunction with the abdominals. For example, the abdominal obliques (Figure 95) stabilize the anterior and lateral portions of the rib cage, providing an important anchor to the origin of the serratus (Figure 96). This anchor allows the serratus to move the scapula on the rib cage rather than working in reverse by elevating, upwardly rotating, and flaring the top eight ribs. The lower fibers of the serratus interdigitate with the abdominal external obliques. Activity of the abdominals encourages activity of the serratus.

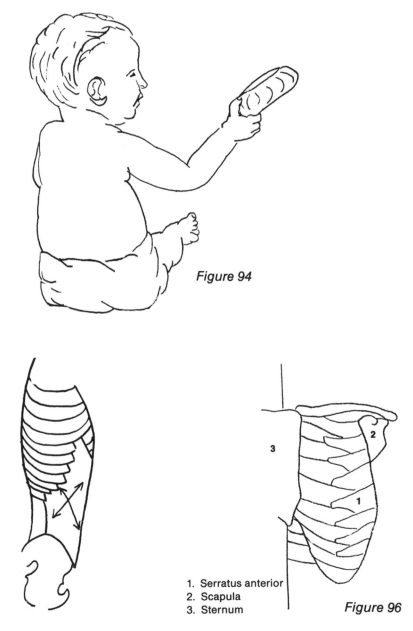

Figure 94

Figure 95

1. Serratus anterior
2. Scapula
3. Sternum

Figure 96

Not only is the serratus anterior used as a mover of the scapula, it also is used to hold the scapula on the rib cage, providing a dynamically fixed origin for the other muscles acting on the humerus. This means that the serratus is holding the scapula and moving it at the same time. Therefore, as the patient reaches, the abdominal obliques prevent the ribs from mechanically following the movement of the arm.

Relationship of abdominals to the total body. The abdominals provide the dynamic connection between the upper and lower portions of the body. The rectus abdominis links the xiphoid process of the sternum with the pubic symphysis (Figure 97). It is a powerful flexor. The abdominal obliques link the lower portion of the rib cage to the pelvis. Between four months and two years of age, as the abdominals develop, the "mushy" or hypotonic appearance of the stomach is progressively replaced with a girdle, creating the curving waist seen in the older child and adult. This girdle connecting trunk and pelvis provides stability for upper extremity function, respiration, stable sitting, and lower extremity control.

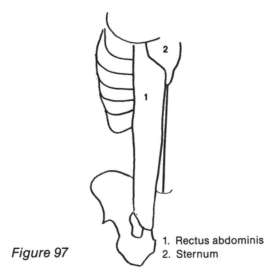

Figure 97

1. Rectus abdominis
2. Sternum

The abdominals indirectly impact on vision as well. Their action on the rib cage provides a base of stability for the shoulder girdle. The shoulders in turn provide a base of stability to the head and neck. As head flexion develops, the eyes follow, moving into a downward gaze. The eyes converge and visual tracking becomes motorically isolated from movement in the rest of the body. Mature occulomotor control allows eyes to move with the head, independent of the head and independent of the direction of movement in the remainder of the body.

Analysis of development

The four-month-old, in prone forearm prop, experiences weight shifting through the shoulder girdle. The child pushes the upper body weight onto one arm (Figure 98). This movement of the upper body over the weight-bearing arm changes the relationship of the arm to the torso. The arm is no longer in a position of abduction but rather the position of flexion. The child will make an attempt to unweight one arm and reach, though lacking the muscle control to maintain one-arm weight bearing. Instead, the child accidentally rolls (Figure 99). The child rolls over the humerus, lengthening rotator cuff muscles, including the powerful latissimus dorsi, thus reducing the pull of the humerus into internal rotation. Rolling over the arm liberates the arm and shoulder from the torso, allowing an increased range of reach.

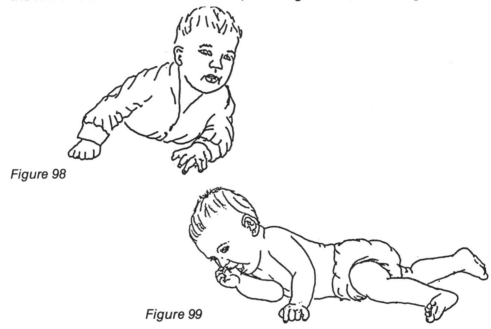

Figure 98

Figure 99

This accidental rolling frightens the four-month-old, who will make many different attempts to control the body in space. As the weight shifts and the child begins to lose control, cervical extension and rotation are used in an attempt to control the fall. This movement takes the child to sidelying, a position that will eventually stimulate lateral head righting and provides important asymmetrical weight bearing, a precursor to lateral mobility and activity through the spine (Figure 100). The child learns to use lateral flexion in the trunk as upper body weight is shifted onto one arm (Figure

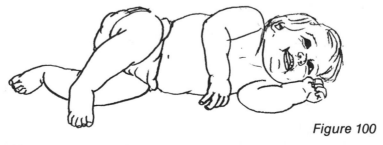

Figure 100

101). Additionally, the child replaces cervical extension and rotation with lateral flexion during the roll and discovers that it is possible to fall into supine rather than stopping in sidelying (Figure 102). These early and initially accidental transitions lead to controlled mobility between the pelvis and shoulder girdle. The child learns to use the latissimus dorsi eccentrically or in its lengthened state.

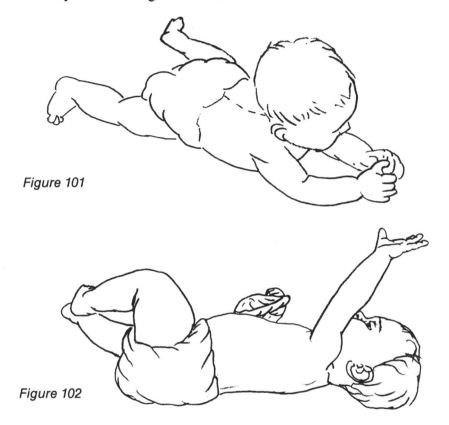

Figure 101

Figure 102

As flexion develops to counterbalance extension, the five-month-old will begin to roll from supine to sidelying with active lateral righting of the head and trunk, elongation of the weight-bearing side, and dissociation of the lower extremities (Figure 103). Because the six-month-old is able to use

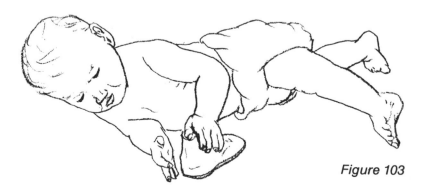

Figure 103

head flexion to initiate the roll, the child can move from supine to sidelying and then to prone. The experience of this early transitional movement and the whole body control that develops with it provides the six-month-old with the arm freedom for social games such as "patty cake" and "so big." The six-month-old also establishes control of the elbow and a fluid unilateral reach. How do all of these wonderful components develop?

The acquisition of unilateral reach. The five-month-old's attempts to control accidental rolling creates a demand on the shoulders that activates muscles, strengthens them and, over time, increases the endurance needed for additional experimentation with upper-extremity-assisted movement. This is an important factor to remember in treatment. Your patient will develop shoulder girdle control as attempts are made to control the movement in and out of prone. Consequently, during treatment, take your patient slightly off balance and encourage returning to the middle (Figure 104).

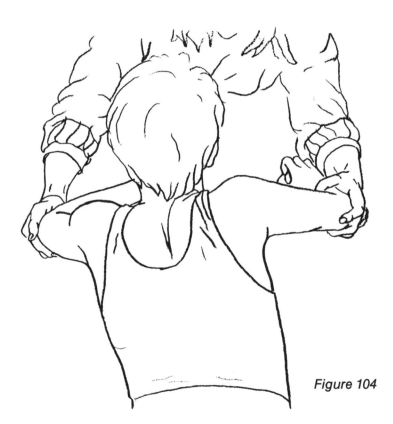

Figure 104

As the five-month-old learns to control balance in prone, the child will acquire enough shoulder girdle control to shift weight to one arm and reach with the unweighted arm (Figure 105). With one humerus and shoulder stabilized in weight bearing and the other mobilized for reach, the two shoulders learn to function independently. The child is then able to use isolated unilateral control of one arm. If this component of development does not occur, the patient will fix strongly with one arm as the other arm is used for function (Figure 106).

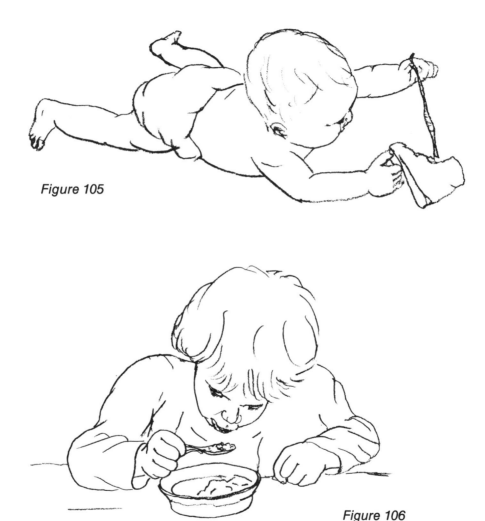

Figure 105

Figure 106

The relationship of elbow to shoulder. The five-month-old prepares for control of elbow extension by lengthening the elbow flexors through hand-to-foot play (Figure 107). Hand-to-foot play allows the child the use of sustained traction to elongate the elbow flexors. We can apply this normal process to treatment by using sustained traction to inhibit elbow flexion spasticity (Figure 108). The five-month-old also pushes up on extended arms, initially fisting the hands to generate proximal power (Figure 109). The function of the elbow is to change the length of the arm. As elbow flexion and extension are used against a surface, the child moves away from and closer to the surface during play (Figure 110).

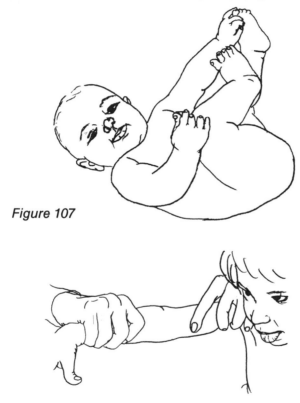

Figure 107

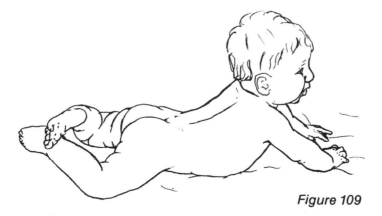

Figure 108

Figure 109

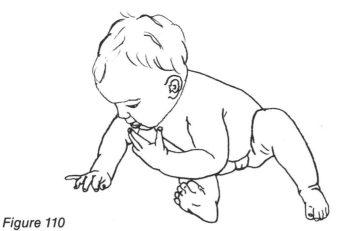

Figure 110

Adults, as well as children, use the elbows to help move off of the floor, out of bed, and out of a chair. Patients with movement limitations in gait use elbow extension to help utilize crutches and walkers. We use the whole arm in weight bearing as we unweight our pelvis and hips, making a transition possible. However, even with full elbow extension, the arm is not long enough to accomplish pelvic unweighting on its own. Consequently, the clavicle depresses the shoulders to give us additional arm length (Figure 111). The latissimus dorsi supports this action by pulling the shoulder girdle down. It works with the elbow during transfer and ambulation with aides (Sieg and Adams 1985). Thus extended arm-weight shifting, in a variety of positions, will lead to shoulder girdle depression.

Assessment and treatment of the trunk for wide range reach
Lack of head and neck control will interfere with reach above ninety degrees. Many patients initiate movement and attempt to control posture with head and neck hyperextension and tongue retraction (Figure 112).

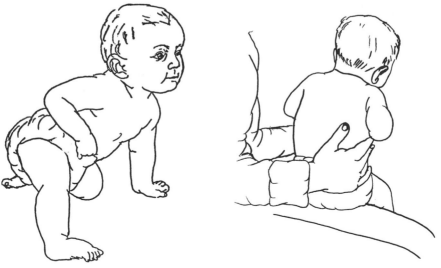

Figure 111   *Figure 112*

This pattern moves the patient's upper body behind the center of gravity. In an attempt to prevent a fall, the shoulders elevate to stabilize the head and neck. In addition, the shoulders will protract to bring the body in line with gravity. With compensatory shoulder protraction, the upper arms are usually held in adduction, extension, and internal rotation. Furthermore, asymmetry is used to gain postural stability. This adaptation to normal postural control prevents the shoulders from obtaining the proper position and relationship to the torso. When the shoulders are involved in compensatory asymmetrical elevation and protraction, they will be unavailable for functional overhead reach.

Techniques to free up the shoulders from the head and neck are described in Chapter 3. Facilitation of head and neck, and control of shoulders that are depressed and expanded, will ultimately improve range and quality of reach (Figures 113-115). You are stabilizing the shoulders and progressively moving your patient's torso off center. Wait for the head and neck to right themselves. This response may take one or two minutes. Give it

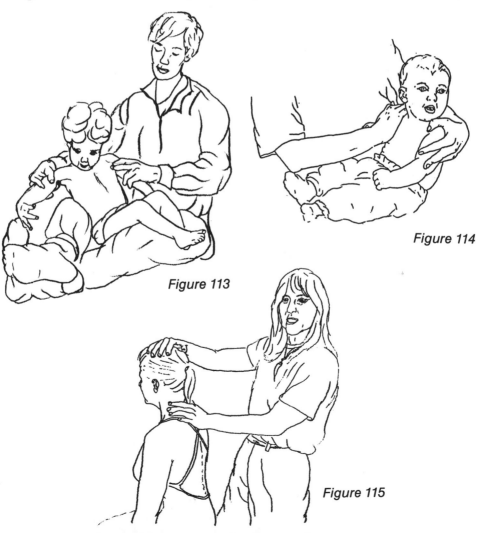

Figure 113

Figure 114

Figure 115

time. You can help the torso follow the righting response of the head and neck. However, treatment for head and neck control may not be adequate because the oral mechanism is involved in this dysfunctional pattern of movement. A habitual force of head and neck hyperextension with tongue retraction potentially leads to retraction of the lips and cheeks with extension and retraction of the jaw (Alexander 1987). Providing your patient with graded pressure input to the cheeks, lips, and tongue will improve the sensorimotor base for oral control (Figure 116). Your input elongates lip and cheek musculature, providing greater range and ease of oral movements. Carryover of oral control to feeding and phonation will help establish this improved oral control as the head and neck work more efficiently off the shoulder girdle.

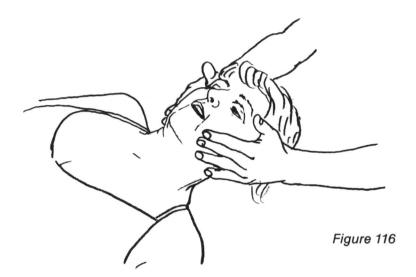

Figure 116

As your patient attempts to reach above the head without the control of the spine or support of abdominal obliques, the compensatory patterns that result can be counterproductive to wide-range reach as well as whole-body movements. The most typical adaptation is the use of the rectus abdominis to stabilize the front of the body. The use of this muscle without support from the abdominal obliques generates a strong pull of the sternum toward the base of the pubis. This forces the patient to be dominated by generalized postural flexion. This will limit the anterior elongation needed for prone function, controlled sitting, and transitional movement patterns. By the nature of its downward and inward pull on the sternum, an unopposed rectus abdominis will restrict the movement of the ribs during respiration and phonation and will result in flattening of the thoracic cavity (Figure 117). Therefore, when your patient uses the rectus abdominis, there will be a lack of anterior-vertical freedom between the shoulders and pelvis. Moreover, the ability of the shoulders to expand on the rib cage will be restricted. Elongation of the rectus abdominis and facilitation of obliques will be a key factor in the acquisition of humeral range and the development of postural control.

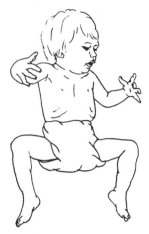

Figure 117

Elongation of rectus abdominis as you facilitate overhead reach can be accomplished in all positions. In normal development this muscle is lengthened in forearm prop and further lengthened in extended-arm weight bearing. As described in Chapter 3, the techniques designed to gain extension of the lumbar spine also will serve to lengthen the rectus abdominis. However, to ensure that your inhibition has an impact directly on the muscle, be certain that you or the weight-bearing surface has maximum contact with the muscle. You can stabilize the area of origin (tip of sternum and lower ribs) and insertion (base of pubis) as you lengthen the anterior portion of the trunk (Figures 118-120). It is possible to inhibit the whole length of the muscle with a deep graded pressure through a slow,

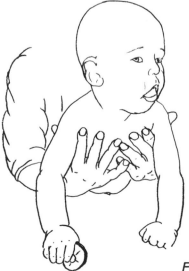

Figure 118

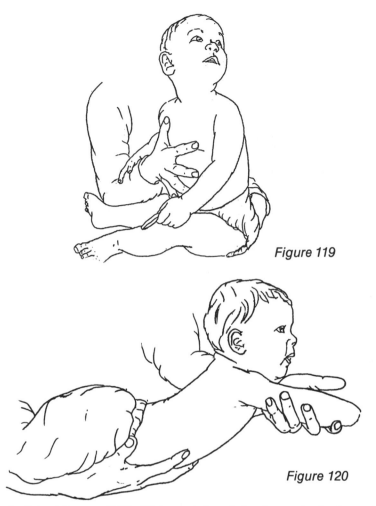

Figure 119

Figure 120

controlled slide (Figure 121). This myofascial release technique (Barnes 1986) follows the same principles as inhibition. You are waiting for a "give" or softening of the muscle tone and surrounding tissue, a signal that you can move the patient into a greater range.

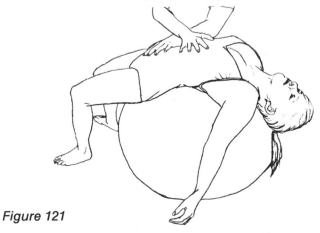

Figure 121

As your patient uses the rectus abdominis to stabilize the anterior portion of the body, the latissimus dorsi often will be used to stabilize the posterior portion. When acting on the arm, the latissimus dorsi will internally rotate, adduct, and extend the humerus. This muscle is designed to symmetrically flex the trunk or hyperextend the lumbar spine depending upon the body's relationship to the center of gravity (see Appendix C). When working unilaterally the latissimus can laterally flex the trunk.

When your patient attempts to use the latissimus dorsi as compensation for lack of abdominal obliques, the latissimus will draw the shoulder girdle down and toward a hiked or elevated pelvis (Figure 122). This shortening of the trunk restricts lateral and diagonal weight shifting and postural reactions in all positions. A restricted or poorly controlled latissimus dorsi can dominate the posture of the shoulder by pulling the humerus into extension and internal rotation. It also restricts the upward rotation of the scapula by binding its inferior border to the lower three or four ribs.

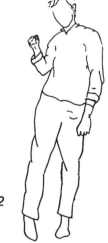

Figure 122

Facilitation techniques that encourage lateral weight shifting will lengthen the latissimus dorsi and foster eccentric activity. This can be accomplished in sideyling (Figure 123), prone (Figure 124), or sitting (Figure 125). With your guidance, the patient's own movement may be enough to inhibit dysfunctional tone.

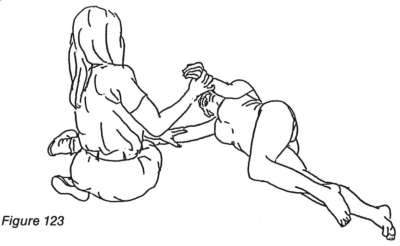

Figure 123

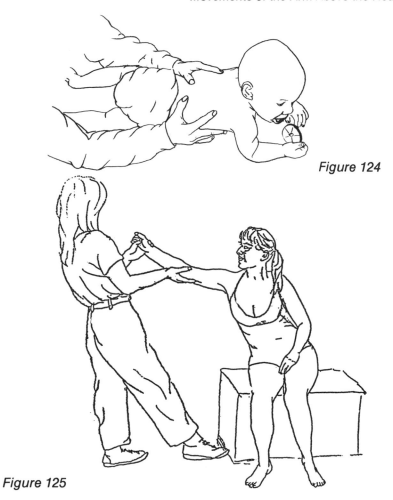

Figure 124

Figure 125

When indirect methods of intervention are not sufficient, you can directly lengthen the latissimus dorsi using the same handling approach described for the rectus abdominis. Your direct contact with the latissimus dorsi can have a dramatic effect on the whole body as well as the range of humeral reach. Your hands travel the length of the muscle, from the iliac crest through the axilla. Because the muscle insertion in the anterior portion of the humerus is usually quite tight, your input into the axilla will need strategic grading. Direct treatment of the latissimus can be managed in sidelying where bilateral traction is applied to the weight-bearing arm and leg (Figure 126). Treatment can also be accomplished in sidelying, where

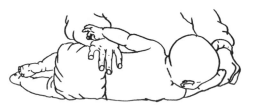

Figure 126

a slow, controlled slide is applied to the non-weight-bearing side (Figure 127) (Barnes 1987). You can inhibit the dysfunctional muscle activity of the latissimus dorsi in sitting with rotation of the spine (Figure 128). It is important to point out here that the majority of trunk rotation occurs in the thoracic spine. Approximately 70 degrees of axial rotation is available in the thorax whereas a maximum of 10 degrees is available in the lumbar spine (Kapandji 1974). Consequently, when you facilitate trunk rotation, your force is on the rib cage between T-8 and T-12 with the pelvis stabilized. Furthermore, it would be inappropriate to use the shoulders as a key point of control for rotation because you risk shifting the shoulders over the spine rather than obtaining true spinal rotation.

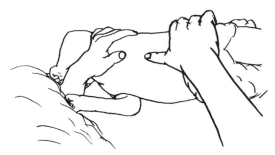

Figure 127

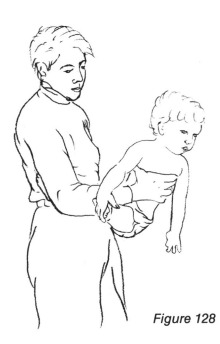

Figure 128

As you progressively manage the tight rectus abdominis and latissimus dorsi, you will want to prepare the rib cage for facilitation of abdominal obliques. Because the alignment of the rib cage is essential for shoulder stability and abdominal activity, your hand contact will draw the ribs in the direction of the feet (Figure 129). You will visualize the ribs moving freely from each other. Your hands will systematically make contact with all aspects of the ribs. The anterior plane, where the ribs attach to the sternum (Figure 130) and the posterior and lateral planes near the ribs' attachment to the spine (Figure 131) will benefit from direct intervention. The ribs are designed to move up and down, as well as in and out. Furthermore, these movements consist of upward and downward axial rotation. Deep pressure, traction, and graded movement allow the patient a feeling of stability as you inhibit the muscle tone and gain range. Facilitating

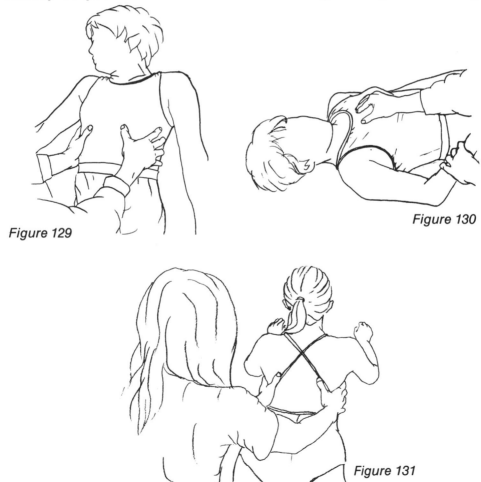

Figure 129

Figure 130

Figure 131

abdominal obliques can be accomplished with prone weight shifting where the abdominals will stabilize against the weight-bearing surface (Figure 132). In quadruped the weight is shifted diagonally (Figure 133). In supine the lower body weight is shifted diagonally with the patient returning the legs to the middle (Figure 134). Appendix C will reinforce your understanding of the role of the abdominals in whole-body movement.

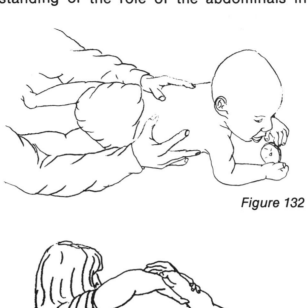

Figure 132

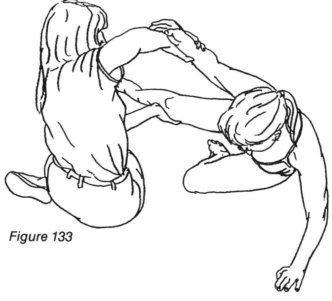

Figure 133

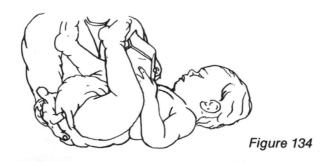

Figure 134

Assessment and treatment of shoulder and arm to support reach

The patient with poor lumbar extension will tend to use scapular adduction to support postural control. Over time, the consistent and strong overuse of the trapezius and rhomboids will interfere with the upward rotation of the scapula, needed for overhead reach. You can move the scapula slowly into upward rotation, maintaining deep pressure contact along the medial and inferior border (Figures 135-136). Another option is to stabilize the lateral aspect of the ribs and slowly move the arm and shoulder in progressively larger ranges of flexion and abduction (Figure 137). It is

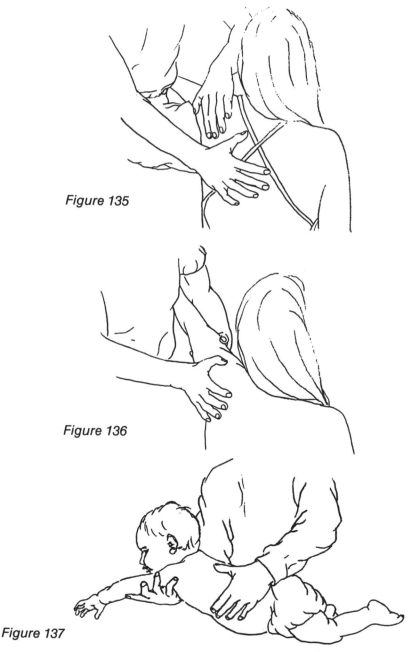

Figure 135

Figure 136

Figure 137

important to follow specific treatment strategies with facilitation that encourages the patient to use the new range independently (Figure 138).

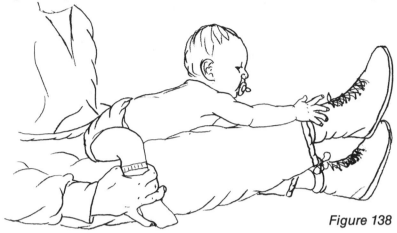

Figure 138

We now understand the importance of developing specialized activity of one shoulder independent of the other in order to develop a unilateral reach. When your patient fails to establish this movement component independently, you may slowly bring one shoulder forward with the other arm in weight bearing (Figure 139). Your end goal is to move one arm and shoulder forward in this same position (Figure 140). Remember to follow up with active use of this shoulder range (Figure 141) and continue facilitation of prone weight shifting.

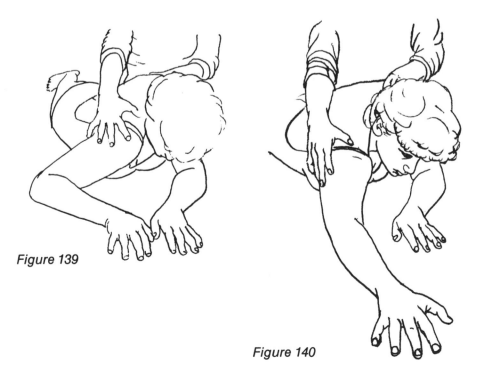

Figure 139

Figure 140

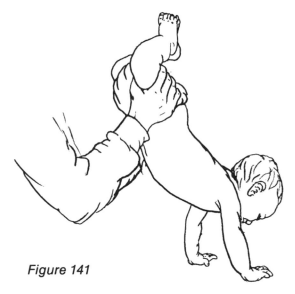

Figure 141

Many patients lack active and strong elbow extension for protective responses and transitional movements. Because the elbow is a middle joint, it is somewhat at the mercy of the humerus and wrist, just as the knee depends on hip and foot control. Facilitation of elbow extension against a surface stimulates the strength and endurance needed for midrange control (concentric and eccentric grading of elbow flexors and extensors). Elbow extension with reach is often gravity-assisted and does not, in and of itself, create the demand needed for the full development of elbow control. Facilitation from side prop to side sit will create the proper demand. In the side prop position, your patient's weight-bearing arm should be internally rotated, with the hand close to the trunk (Figure 142).

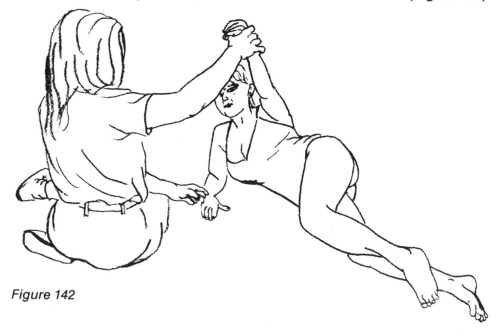

Figure 142

This hand placement ensures that the length of the arm will be adequate to take the patient into full sit. You can stabilize the patient's hand as you initiate the anterior, diagonal lift (Figure 143). You are shifting the patient's weight toward the weight-bearing hand. It is important that you avoid executing the lift for the patient. Begin the lift and wait for your patient to respond. Lateral weight shifting in quadruped also will challenge the elbows (Figure 144). Weight bearing with the arms behind the rib cage will stimulate elbow and humeral extension for backward protective responses (Figure 145).

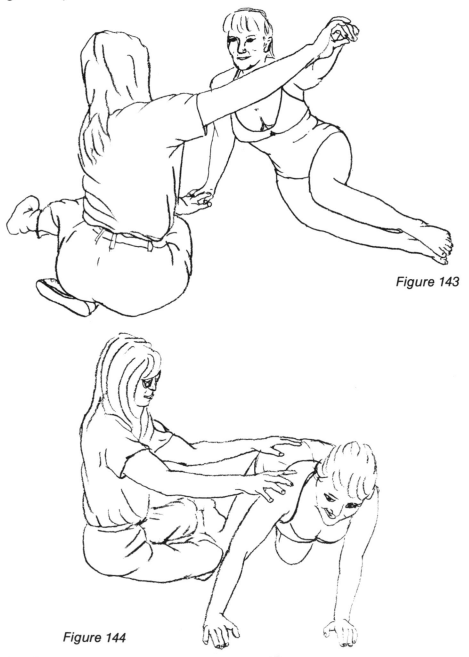

Figure 143

Figure 144

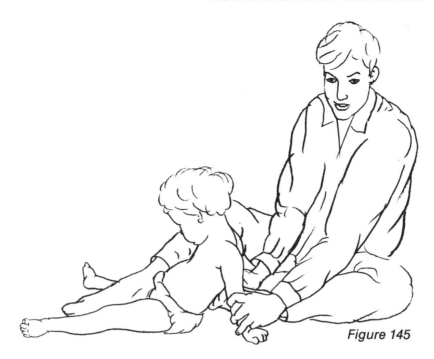

Figure 145

Treatment for humeral rotation

Like the elbow, facilitating controlled humeral rotation is most effective when treatment takes place during transitional movement patterns. As the torso moves over and around a humerus that is stabilized in weight bearing, the rotational relationship between arm and trunk changes. For example, the arm in sidelying can be in neutral rotation (Figure 146) and,

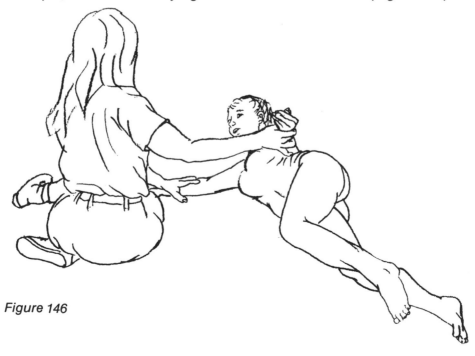

Figure 146

as the patient moves into side prop, the arm moves into external rotation (Figure 147). With that in mind, you will concentrate on facilitation, in upper extremity weight bearing, around the body axis (Figures 148-151). You are helping the body move over and around the arm. As rotational control develops in transitions, you can facilitate it in reach.

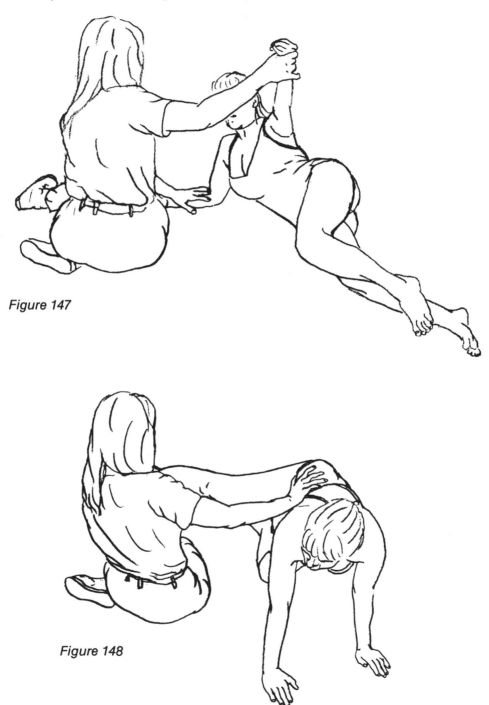

Figure 147

Figure 148

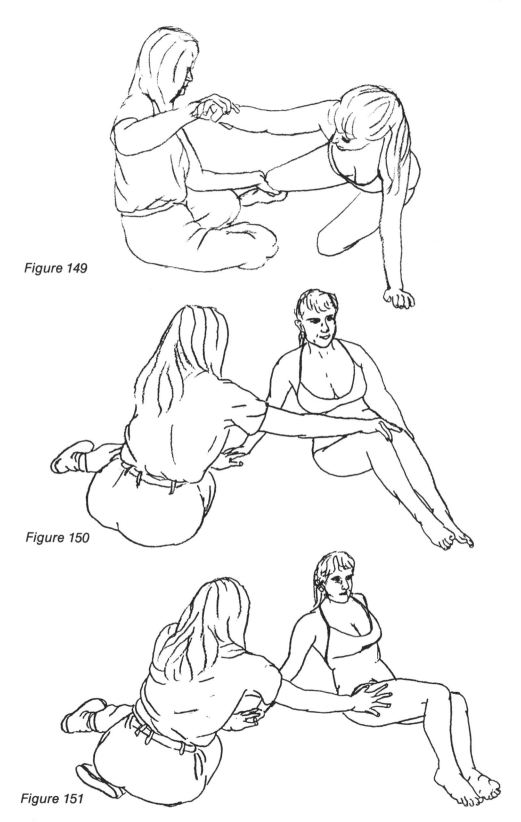

Figure 149

Figure 150

Figure 151

Summary

The treatment approaches described in the last two chapters will promote functional use of the arm for reach and weight bearing. Consequently, during treatment you are conducting an ongoing assessment of your patient's independent range of reach, ability of the arm to maintain its posture in space, and the arm's control as it follows a moving object. You also will consistently ask your patient to use the arms in transitions without the assistance of your hands.

Observe the whole-body movements of your patient with an analytical eye. What movements can he do independently and efficiently? What can be done with your assistance? What movement patterns are impossible? Identify the components of movement that are missing from your patient's movement repertoire. Inhibit the abnormal muscle tone interfering with the execution of the movement pattern. Facilitate part or all of the movement pattern by (1) helping the patient maintain the proper alignment and relationship to the center of gravity, (2) guiding the speed and excursion of the movement, (3) inhibiting inefficient, habituated patterns as they are being used, (4) telling the patient when the movement looks better, and (5) allowing the patient time to experience the improved movement without the support of your hands.

Be open to the communication coming from the patient's body. It is trying to tell you what it needs. Allow treatment to be a spontaneous, creative process for both you and the patient. Remember that therapy is a graceful and fluid interaction between two people, each sharing the control.

References

Alexander, R. 1987. Respiratory and oral-motor functioning. In *Therapeutic exercise in developmental disabilities,* edited by B. Connolly and P. Montgomery. Tennessee: Chattanooga Corporation.

Barnes, J. 1986. Myofascial Release Seminar I. Chicago, IL.

———. 1987. Myofascial Release Seminar II. Captiva, FL.

Kapandji, I. 1982. *The physiology of the joints,* Vol. 3. New York: Churchill Livingstone.

———. 1974. *The physiology of the joints,* Vol. I. New York: Churchill Livingstone.

Sieg, K., and S. Adams. 1985. *Illustrated essentials of musculoskeletal anatomy.* Gainesville, FL: Mega Books.

CHAPTER 5

Treatment for Basic Hand Function

The way to conquer the dysfunctional hand is to treat it directly, aggressively, with a sound knowledge base, and from a functional perspective.

The Functional Perspective

The functional role of the hand is to shape itself around objects and on top of surfaces. It accomplishes these two functions through dynamic palmar arches and combined movements of the wrist and forearm. This sounds simple enough. But anyone who has attempted to improve the performance of the neurologically impaired hand is well acquainted with the challenge of this task. I have spent years convincing people that my patients' hands were just not ready for function, that more proximal control was needed, more weight-bearing experience was needed, or the scapula was still too unstable. Rationalization is a necessary skill when facing the unknown.

The hand can be powerful. You can shape your hand around an object and completely immobilize it in your palm. You can maintain this powerful grasp when resistance is placed on the object by the nature of its weight or because some force is trying to pull it from you. And yet, at the same time, the hand is a delicate instrument, the tool of the artist or the surgeon. You can place a small object in your palm and move it around delicately within your hand. You have complicated blends of movements in your hand that allow you to button, use scissors, tie shoes, develop economic specialties, and function independently in our highly evolved, tool-using species.

This chapter will provide information on how the hand, wrist, and forearm work together to support upper extremity weight bearing, grasp, and release. The information is divided into many component parts. You will be given specific treatment techniques to achieve basic hand function by facilitating a working relationship between the hand, wrist, and forearm. Practice these techniques on your friends. They will be grateful for the soothing sensory input.

FOREARM ROTATION

Combined movements of the forearm and wrist orient the hand in space, placing it in the proper position to receive an object or accept a weight-bearing surface. The forearm and wrist move the hand to a place where it can be useful and efficient.

Analysis of component parts

In supination, the radius and the ulna lie side by side. The radius is shaped like a crank. The supinator muscle unwinds the forearm while the biceps tractions or pulls it into supination (Figure 152). The biceps brachii is the most powerful rotator and works at maximum efficiency when the elbow is flexed to 90 degrees. The supinators are more powerful than the pronators. Yet supination can be limited by spasticity of the pronator muscles. A gentle oscillation between the ulna and radius will help to inhibit pronator spasticity (Figure 153).

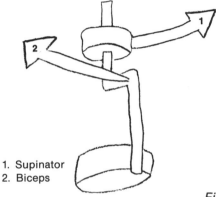

1. Supinator
2. Biceps

Figure 152

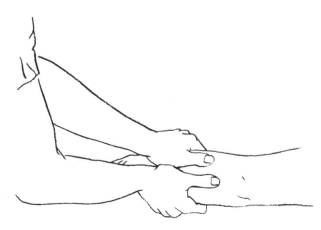

Figure 153

In pronation, the two bones cross each other. The pronator quadratus unwinds the crank or moves radius over ulna, while the pronator teres acts on the radius by tractioning or pulling it (Figure 154). The most functional positions of the forearm are neutral rotation and the degree of pronation seen when writing (Figure 155). Our patients need to develop control of pronation, as well as range into supination (Figure 156).

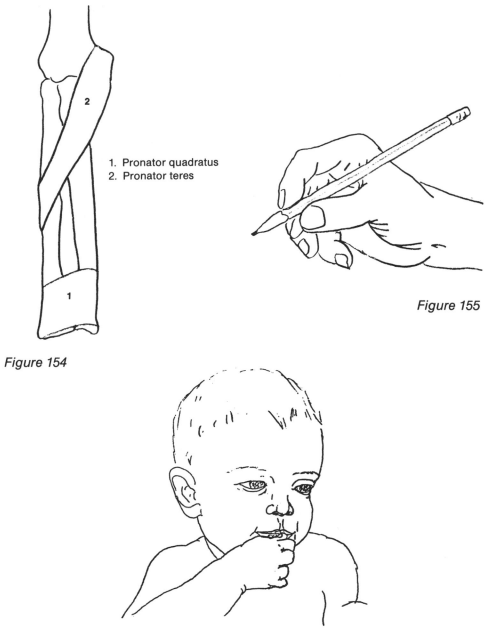

1. Pronator quadratus
2. Pronator teres

Figure 155

Figure 154

Figure 156

Functionally we need control of forearm rotation with the elbow in motion as it is during feeding, tooth brushing, and bathing. We use an ongoing series of rotational movements that continually put the hand in the proper position for function. This series of rotational movements occurs through the ability of the radius to rotate at both ends of the forearm. At its distal end or wrist joint, as the radius rotates, the ulna is displaced through the components of wrist extension and radial deviation. Displacement of the ulna is possible because the ulnar head is not in contact with the carpal bones of the wrist. If your patient's wrist is bound by flexion and ulnar deviation, control of forearm rotation will be blocked.

Rotational movements also occur at the proximal end with the radius rotating on a vertical axis, like a door rotating on a hinge. Again the ulnar head is displaced, but this time the mechanics are made possible by concurrent external rotation of the humerus. When your patient's humerus is bound by a strong pull into internal rotation, control of forearm rotation is again blocked; the door becomes jammed as if the hinges were out of alignment. It becomes obvious that forearm control is dependent on basic control of the humerus and wrist.

To further complicate matters, there is extensive interosseous membrane between the ulna and radius that can become restricted as the spasticity limits the movement of the forearm. This restriction creates problems for the thumb as well as the forearm, since many important thumb extension muscles originate on this tissue. It is helpful to spend some time softening the tissue. A light, gentle, very slow stretch of small areas of the skin, one-third of the forearm at a time, will soften the tissue three-dimensionally, releasing the interosseous membrane as well (Figure 157). Myofascial release techniques (Barnes 1986) work well on restricted forearms.

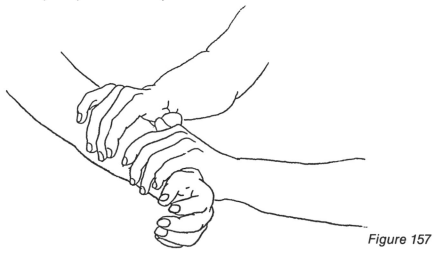

Figure 157

Analysis of development
Early random movements and active swiping will facilitate some essential range of motion and beginning control of the humerus and lower arm. But the systematic way in which the young child develops voluntary control of the forearm is interesting and pertinent information for treatment. For

example, the four-month-old in prone prop will move shoulders, from side to side, over weighted forearms. The forearms are weighted when the elbows are in line with or slightly behind the gleno-humeral joint. The forearms rotate as the lateral weight shifting occurs. The forearm accepting the additional weight will move toward supination, while the other forearm pronates (Figure 158).

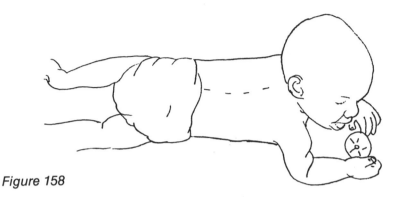

Figure 158

Observe the position of your patients' forearms in prone prop. They often weight bear on elbows and stabilize the position by holding strongly with elbow flexion. As they laterally weight shift, the humerus can easily pivot into internal rotation to mechanically support the upper torso, bypassing important muscle elongation in the mid arm (Figure 159). When you

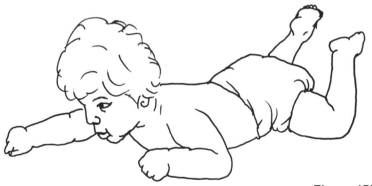

Figure 159

facilitate lateral weight shifting through forearm rotation, you build in this important missing component (Figure 160). You can lengthen the ulnar side of the wrist concurrently by compressing the forearm gently onto the weight-bearing surface as you shift your weight.

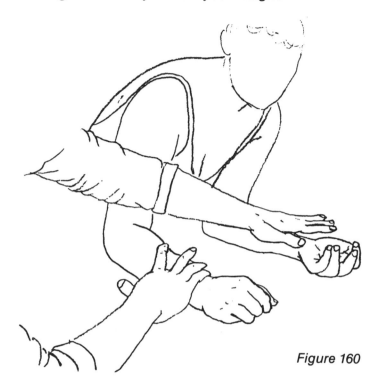

Figure 160

The child at five and six months of age will bring the elbows in front of the gleno-humeral joint, once the forearm muscles are lengthened. The child begins to develop isolated, voluntary control of forearm rotation by working off a humerus stabilized in weight bearing (Figure 161). Thus when treating for forearm control you can stabilize, but not completely immobilize, your patient's humerus (Figure 162).

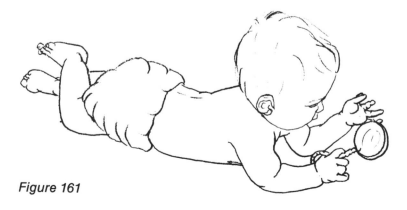

Figure 161

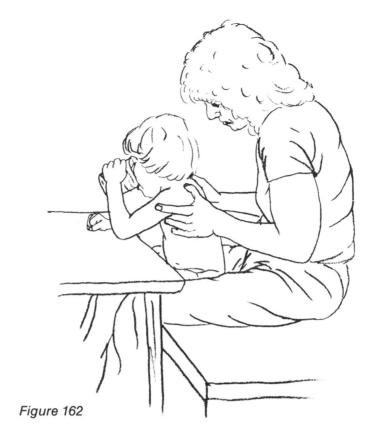

Figure 162

The seven- to eight-month-old child will experiment with forearm rotation in sitting, but will accomplish this by stabilizing the humerus against the rib cage (Figure 163), an approach that is also helpful in treatment. When you stabilize your patient's humerus next to the rib cage, you are preventing the compensatory humeral adduction that is often used in lieu

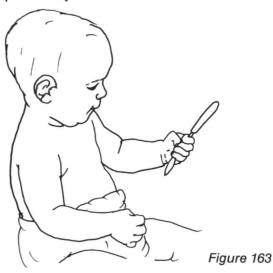

Figure 163

of active forearm rotation (Figure 164). The nine-month-old controls supination with the humerus in any position, as long as the trunk is stable. The child at eleven to twelve months of age controls supination with the humerus in any position. Thus, the normal child will develop voluntary control of the forearm, through successive approximation, over a period of eight months. It will take another twelve months for the child to develop strength for turning knobs and selective mid-range control for self-feeding.

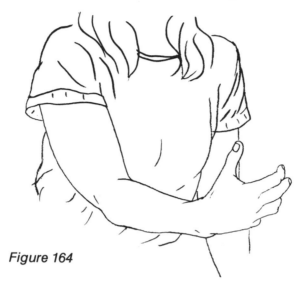

Figure 164

Management of elbow and wrist movement will precede the development of controlled voluntary forearm rotation. However, feel free to stabilize the humerus and gently elongate the ulnar side of the wrist to facilitate forearm rotation (Figure 165). This can be done before your patient develops complete control of the proximal and distal parts. As your patient initially attempts to rotate the forearm, you will feel spurts of supinator activity that in time will become sustained and useful.

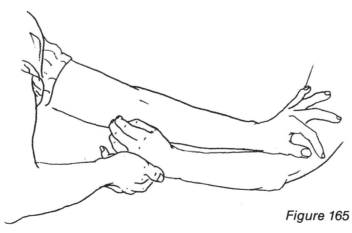

Figure 165

THE WRIST

Flexion and extension

The control of the hand can be viewed from the same perspective as the control of the trunk. In order to manage our bodies in space, we need a balance between flexion and extension in the trunk. When symmetrical flexion and extension work in harmony with each other, we can control our anterior and posterior movements.

For hand function we need that same type of anterior and posterior control of the wrist. With control of symmetrical flexion and extension of the wrist, we are able to hold the wrist in neutral alignment and work the digits from a proximal and dynamically stable point. Symmetrical wrist control comes from the long muscle groups that originate at the distal end of the humerus, cross over the elbow joint, wrist joint and carpals, and insert onto the metacarpals (Figures 166-167).

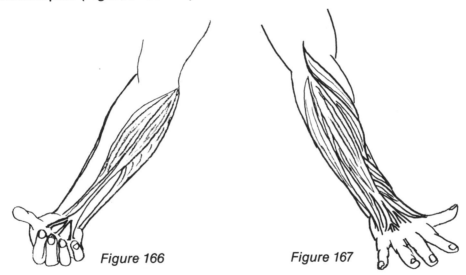

Figure 166   Figure 167

The wrist has greater structural stability when it is in flexion (Tubiana, Thomine, and Mackin 1984). This stability is due to the nature of the capsule and ligamentus structures. This may be one of the reasons for the habitual hand posturing that we observe in patients with neurological disorders.

Radial and ulnar deviation

The body needs lateral control to maintain balance during a lateral weight shift. Lateral control means that the trunk can shorten on one side as the other side of the trunk elongates. Control of lateral movement means that we can shorten on either side and return to the middle.

For hand function we also need control of lateral movements at the wrist. We need ulnar (adduction) and radial (abduction) movement. We need mid-range control of the wrist or the ability to bring the wrist back to the middle.

Analysis of development

The full-term infant's physiological flexion is reflected in the hand as well as in the rest of the body. The child progresses from an asymmetrical grasp where the wrist is flexed and adducted. The grip is not powerful enough to hold an object against resistance (Figure 168). By seven months of age, the child is able to initiate a symmetrical grasp with all digits active and with the wrist straight or in neutral alignment (Figure 169). The symmetry of the wrist accounts for the symmetry of the grasp.

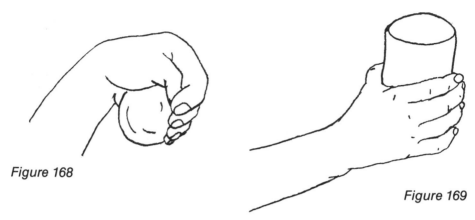

Figure 168

Figure 169

Muscle imbalance around the wrist creates hand dysfunction. When the ulnar side of the wrist is dominated by shortening, the wrist has a tendency to flex. When the wrist is bound by ulnar deviation and flexion, grasp and manipulation are limited because it is mechanically difficult to bring the digits onto the palm (Figure 170). Release is not only easy but is often unavoidable. Elongating the shortened ulnar side will help the patient gain mid-range control of the wrist (Figure 171). Sustaining that elongation

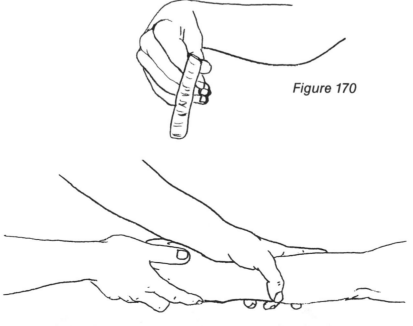

Figure 170

Figure 171

while the patient uses the hand will aid in achieving carryover into function (Figure 172). Weight bearing on the ulnar side of the forearm will help maintain the elongation during active hand use (Figure 173).

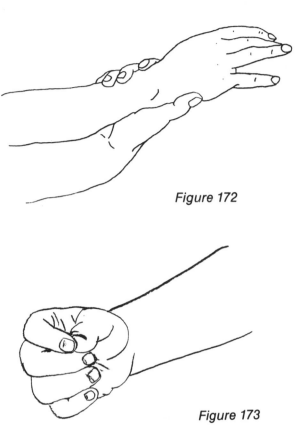

Figure 172

Figure 173

In-depth study and observation of the normal development make us aware of the ongoing relationship between wrist and hand. Wrist and hand tend to develop concurrently, both in and out of weight bearing, because they share many of the same muscles. It becomes impossible, then, to fully describe one without describing the other.

THE HAND

Expansion of the hand

The hand is significantly flexible. It is able to expand or flatten itself during weight bearing. This ability to expand the hand gives the individual a wide base of support for transitional movement patterns. These patterns allow the young child to play on the floor, in and out of a wide variety of positions (Figure 174). It allows the child to explore the environment with minimal effort, before all of the basic movement components and postural reactions are fully developed.

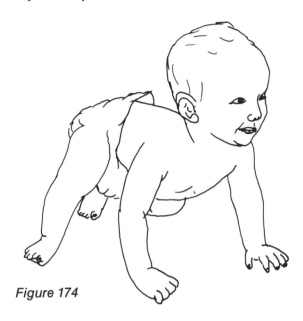

Figure 174

Hand expansion for weight shifting is used throughout life. The adult uses the expanded hand automatically to transfer off the toilet, to protect during an unexpected fall, to straighten out the sheet on a bed, or buff the wax on an automobile.

Therapists use their expanded hands to give their patients the sensory feeling of more controlled movement. When teaching specific therapeutic handling, I often remind the audience to make their hands large, to direct the sensory information through the palms as well as the surfaces of the digits (Figure 175).

As you may have guessed, I think expansion of the hand is an important functional component. It requires joint mobility, joint alignment, and flexibility of the wrist and hand musculature, ligaments, and fascia. Active expansion requires cooperative muscle action. Hand expansion is a prerequisite to grasp, manipulation, and release.

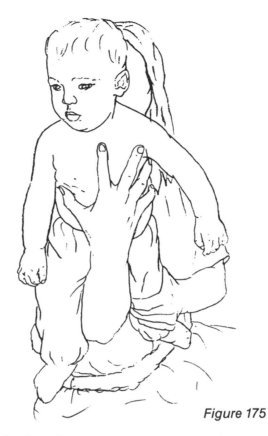

Figure 175

Overexpansion in the hand

In most people, the hand never completely flattens and, from what I understand, it is not supposed to become a pancake. During weight bearing, the hand expands only enough to make contact with the thenar eminence, hypothenar eminence, metacarpal heads, and palmar surfaces of the phalanges (Figure 176). However, I have found greater expansion than this in many normal adults and children. These individuals are usually slightly hypotonic. During weight shift, they often lack enough proximal and distal stability for controlled, slow-motion movement. Once the hands and arms are loaded with partial body weight, they have difficulty holding a posture in mid movement. I enjoy demonstrating this phenomenon on participants in workshops. During slow facilitation of movement, the slightly low-toned therapist makes unusual faces, grunting sounds, and has a tendency toward slight drooling. So much for the sensitive instructor image.

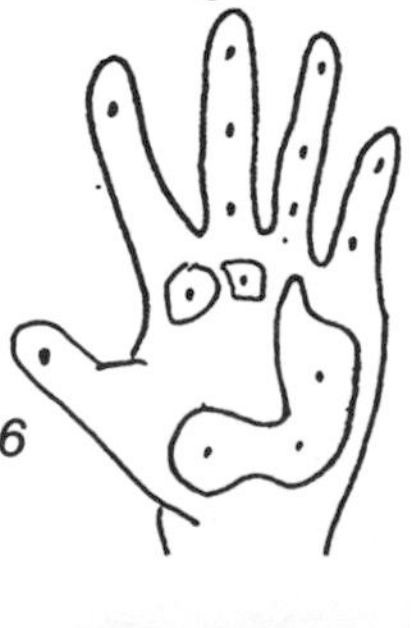

Figure 176

Restricted expansion of the hand
In cerebral palsy, adult hemiplegia, and traumatic head injuries, the patient's hand may not have the natural capability to expand. The expansion may be bound up by spasticity, with the wrist, palm, and digits dominated by marked flexion (Figure 177). Muscles either never elongate or lose their elongation, placing the hand at risk for deformities and skin breakdown. Consistent tight posturing of the hand pulls the joints out of their normal alignment. When spasticity is strong, random and voluntary movements are absent or significantly limited. Obtaining expansion in the patient's hand will reduce abnormal muscle tone and improve the potential for functional hand patterns.

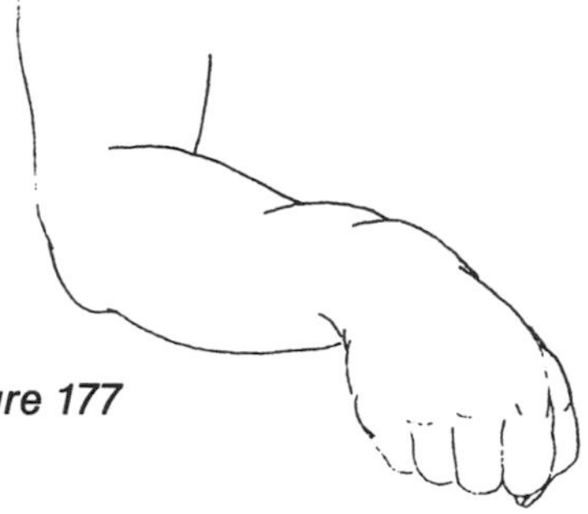

Figure 177

The development of expansion and its relationship to treatment
We learn a great deal about treatment by analyzing the ways in which the child develops an expanded and malleable hand. For example, five- to seven-month-old chidren shift weight laterally through their hands as they support themselves prone on extended arms, supported sit, and in quadruped. This helps expand the width of the hand and lengthen the long finger flexors that cross over the wrist as well as lengthening the lateral aspects of the wrist. Facilitating a lateral movement of the body over the extended arms will help expand the width of your patient's hand (Figure 178).

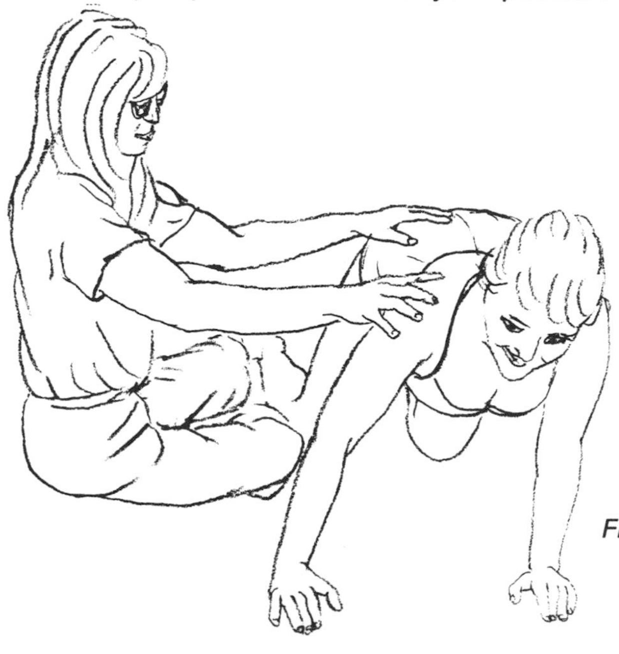

Figure 178

You can directly expand the width of your patient's hand by using a firm graded squeeze with a generalized deep oscillating massage between the hypothenar eminence and the thenar eminence (Figure 179). This technique helps relax the tightly fisted hand and adducted thumb. The degree of pressure you use is similar to the deep pressure felt in weight bearing. However, you will be applying the pressure into the dorsal as well as the palmar surfaces. The pressure into the palmar surface is slightly greater than the dorsal pressure, to avoid the complete flattening of the hand. This deep pressure is felt through the skin, into the deep tissue and joints. Firm handling with slow graded movement inhibits spasticity and facilitates sensory awareness. Maintaining a neutral wrist position as you inhibit the muscle tone will place the long finger flexors and extensors in a better position for balanced activity.

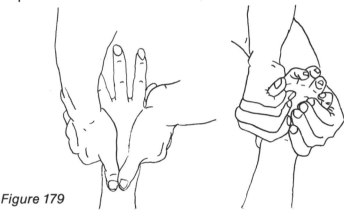

Figure 179

The six- to eight-month-old child rocks back and forth in quadruped, expanding the hand in a longitudinal plane. The long finger flexors slowly become lengthened over the wrist and through the palm. Facilitating an anterior and posterior weight shift in patients who can take support on extended arms will help expand the length of their hands (Figure 180).

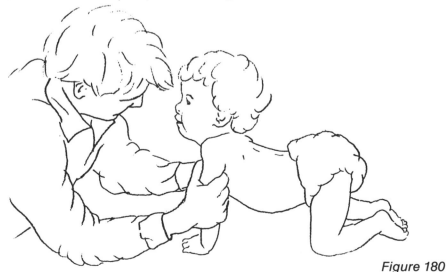

Figure 180

You can expand the length of the hand by gently shortening the patient's long finger extensors with your thumb. The long finger flexors are lengthened by gently tractioning them toward the distal portion of the hand (Figure 181). Again, you will be exerting firm, graded pressure. Maintaining lengthwise expansion is difficult in the hand dominated by flexion. Again, it is best to begin with the wrist in neutral and very slowly move into wrist extension. Facilitating weight bearing after you use this treatment technique will improve carryover.

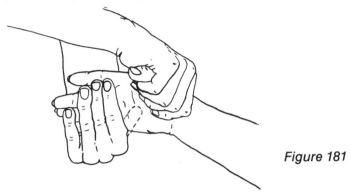

Figure 181

The eight- to twelve-month-old child moves from sitting to quadruped and back to sitting again. This transitional movement creates a diagonal shift of weight through the hand. It expands the hand in an oblique direction, making opposition possible. The weight shift also elongates the web space, creating more room for objects during grasp. The weight-bearing input stimulates active stabilization by the thumb. Diagonal weight shifting on extended arms can be facilitated in therapy to gain an oblique expansion in the hand (Figure 182). Oblique expansion will reduce the pull of the thumb into the palm as the patient attempts to grasp.

You can expand the hand in a diagonal direction by combining deep, angular, oscillating pressure (Figure 183). You can capture the patient's thumb from the base to the distal joint. Small movements of the thumb will inhibit abnormal muscle tone. Gentle traction at the base of the thumb will further inhibit spasticity and help realign the joints (Figure 184).

Expansion of the hand takes the normal child five to six months. The hands are bombarded by partial body weight and active, controlled movement during play. The child moves body weight over a hand that is stabilized by the surface. With treatment, maintained expansion of the spastic hand will take time. Many patients cannot tolerate transitional movements needed for hand expansion. Some patients have not developed the postural reactions needed to move in and out of positions. The hand may be too tightly fisted to accept weight without discomfort. Moreover, playing with movement in and out of quadruped is often an inappropriate approach for the older patient. Expansion of the hand cannot wait until the patient is ready for weight bearing. It is productive to expand the hand directly.

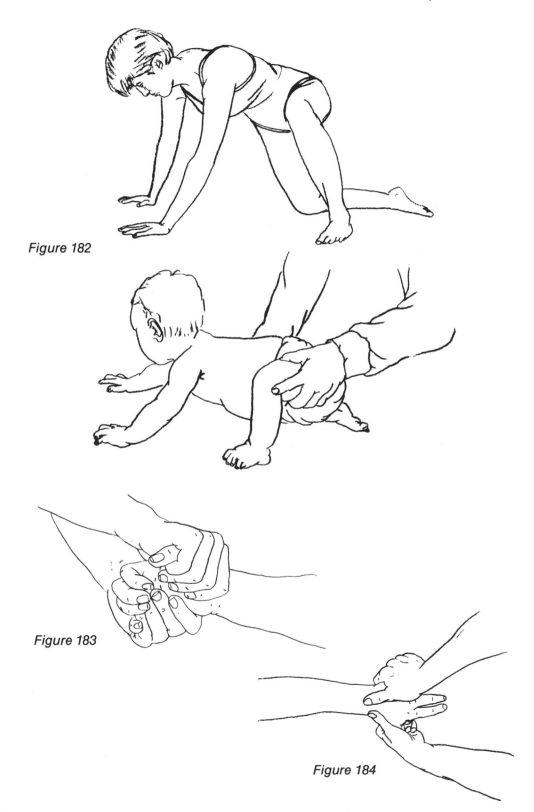

Figure 182

Figure 183

Figure 184

Maintaining the expansion in weight bearing

You can hold the expansion in the hand and bring the patient into weight bearing on top of your hand as you gradually lengthen the long finger flexors that cross over the wrist (Figure 185). As the patient's hand is loaded with the body weight, you can withdraw your hand. As you maintain the wrist close to a 90-degree angle, spasticity will be inhibited by the nature of the weight-bearing position. With the wrist perpendicular to the hand,

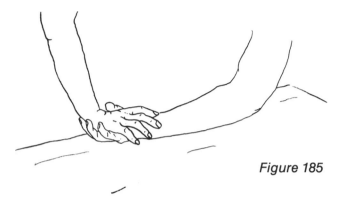

Figure 185

the weight is distributed equally through the palm and digits. As the angle of the wrist changes, the distribution of the weight also changes. For example, when the wrist angle is less than 90 degrees, the distribution of weight through the hand shifts toward the heel of the hand, unweighting the fingers (Figure 186). This wrist angle allows the abnormal muscle tone to be expressed in the digits.

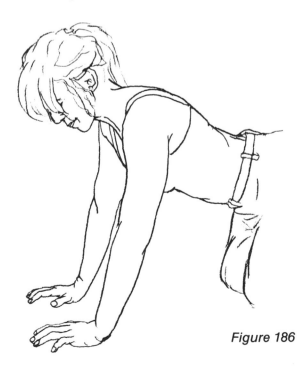

Figure 186

A partially expandable hand can benefit from weight bearing over a roll (Figure 187). There will be equal weight distribution through the hand over the contour of the weight-bearing surface. Weight bearing onto a contoured surface, in and of itself, will help to expand the hand and inhibit dysfunctional muscle tone.

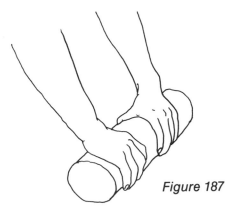

Figure 187

Facilitating wrist extension with palmar expansion will help your patient begin to combine wrist and hand components. Allow the hand to rest comfortably on a table where the patient can work wrist extensors off a stable surface (Figure 188). Light compression of the radius and ulna will inhibit abnormal tone in the forearm.

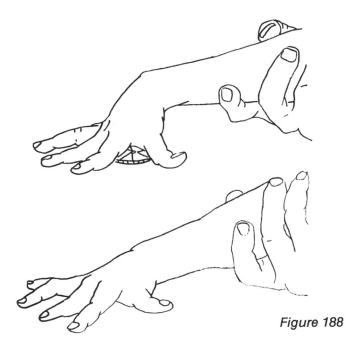

Figure 188

Understanding associated reactions

The inability to maintain expansion of the hand may be due to the influence of associated reactions. Associated reactions are atypical postures that occur with the effort of movement, oral communication, or an emotional response. The motor expression of the atypical posture is fairly consistent regardless of the type of stimulus (effort) that initiated it (Figure 189). In other words, it always looks the same. Once the effortful situation is over,

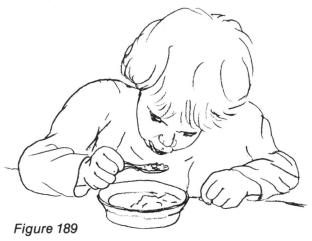

Figure 189

there will be continued evidence of the increased muscle tone for a few additional moments. Associated reactions put the extremity at an anatomical risk and interfere with expansion of the hand. Associated reactions can be reduced with treatment, but they never completely disappear. It is best to inhibit this abnormal reaction in the circumstance that initiates it (Figure 190).

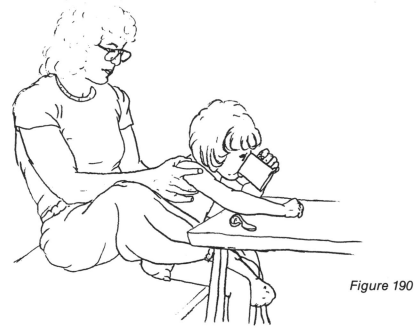

Figure 190

Associated movements

An associated reaction is different than an associated movement. Associated movements mirror the motor effort (Figure 191). If a patient points with the right index finger, the left index finger will also extend. Associated movements disappear as soon as the effort has ended.

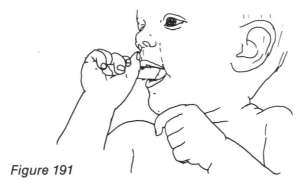

Figure 191

Associated movements are normal reactions to effort and unfamiliar situations. Except in rare genetic cases, they do not interfere with expansion. Most associated movements will lessen with central nervous system maturity.

Shaping of the hand through palmar arches

The normal hand expands to shape itself on a weight-bearing surface. It also expands to shape itself around objects. Erhardt (1982) calls this adaptation "accommodation." This is a wonderful adjective because it gives us a visualization of how flexible and responsive the hand can be. The hand is capable of an infinite variety of both simple and complex motor patterns. These functional hand patterns are created through a blending of movements of the forearm, wrist, palm, and digits. Movement blends allow the hand to shape itself for palpation, grasp, manipulation, and release.

Analysis of component parts

The movement possibilities of the hand are a result of a complex anatomical and kinesiological structure. There are nineteen bones, seventeen gliding articulating surfaces, nineteen muscles and tendons that are activated in the forearm (Tubiana, Thomine, and Mackin 1984). To feel this forearm activity, place your hand lightly around your mid forearm. Wiggle your fingers slightly and you will feel the activity of the long finger flexors and extensors.

Proximal control of the hand is based, in part, on the palmar arches. Therefore, what the fingers do is a reflection of what the palm is doing. The palm is made up of three types of arches.

The TRANSVERSE or carpal arch is formed by the metacarpal heads and distal row of carpal bones (Tubiana, Thomine, and Mackin 1984). This arch allows our hands to shape into a gutter (Figure 192). It traverses or runs the width of the hand and brings the ulnar and radial borders of the hand

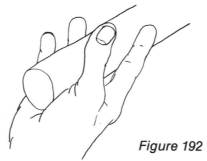

Figure 192

toward each other. When the arch is expanded, the hand is wider or broader. Tightly flexed thumbs may block the development or use of this arch. When the arch is expanded, the hand is wider or broader.

The LONGITUDINAL or carpometacarpo-phalangeal arches fan out from the wrist and are concave on the palmar surfaces (Kapandji 1982). In its simplest form, these arches support a basic cylindrical grasp (Figure 193). When the arches are expanded, the hand is longer.

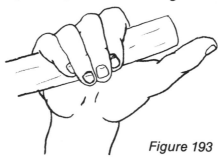

Figure 193

The OBLIQUE arches link the thumb to each of the finger tips for opposition (Figure 194). The arches run diagonally through the hand. When these arches are expanded, the hand is large with the fingers abducted and the thumb extended.

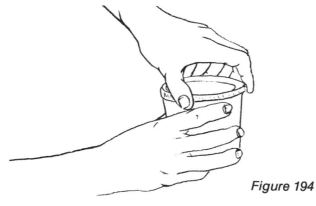

Figure 194

The relationship of expansion to palmar arches
Expansion of the hand and palmar arches develops simultaneously as the young child moves in and out of a variety of positions on extended arms, transferring body weight over hands stabilized against a supporting surface. As the child's center of gravity changes, the fingers cling to the supporting surface in an attempt to prevent a loss of balance (Figure 195).

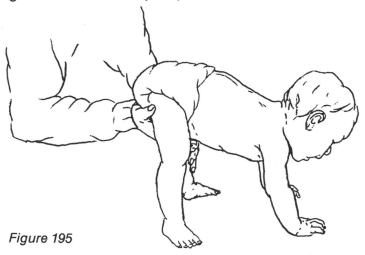

Figure 195

As the fingers cling to the surface, the arches develop. Arches are a component of balance reactions, both in the hands and in the feet. Keep in mind that the normal child repeats these sensorimotor experiences an infinite number of times. Successful treatment for palmar arches will take time and many repetitions. In addition, you will need to attend to your patient's wrist control as you facilitate hand function.

The development of grasp and its relationship to treatment
The symmetrical grasp allows us to embed an object in the palm and flex all the digits around it (Figure 196). This palmar grip orientation immobilizes an object within the hand. In order to move the object, the movement must take place at the wrist, arm, or trunk. This type of hand pattern gives us a powerful grasp. Power in the hand develops before precision.

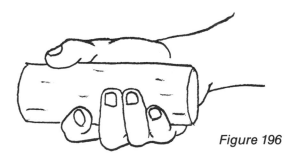

Figure 196

The normal child from birth to three months will experience graceful and varied hand patterns during random movements (Figure 197). Random movements reduce the influence of physiological flexion. The breastfed infant uses the hands to "milk" mom's breasts during feeding through an automatic flexion-and-extension pattern. Many young infants also manage to find their thumbs for sucking.

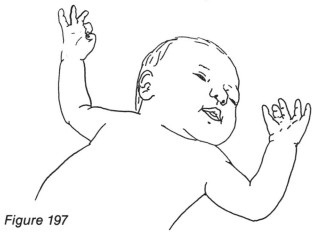

Figure 197

By three months of age, the child will reach toward immediately available objects and, with help, manage to trap them in the ulnar side of the palm (Figure 198). By four months, the child has already realized the value of hands, engaging in hand-on-body contact (Figure 199) and hand-to-object contact. This hand contact is initially performed without the ability to grade the pressure. Consequently, the child squeezes the objects hard. The ungraded pressure shapes the hand around the form.

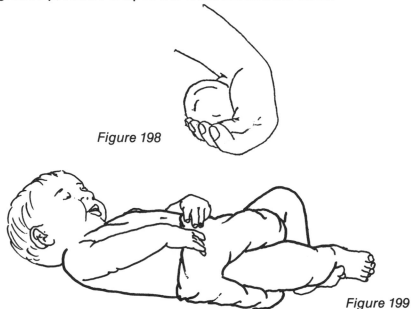

Figure 198

Figure 199

By five months, the child is developing increased success at touching and grabbing objects, with greater symmetry seen in the digits. The object is held with all the fingers participating and the thumb actively adducting against the object as well (Figure 200). At this time, the grasp lacks power because the wrist is still dominated by flexion.

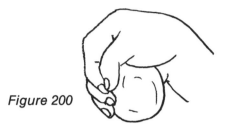

Figure 200

The child establishes a basic palmar grip on varying shaped objects during the sixth and seventh months, a grip which Erhardt (1982) calls the radial-palmar grasp. The wrist is straight, the arches are active, and the thumb is properly opposed (Figure 201). However, the child often drops the object as the arm is straightened. The child needs to find a way to hold a grip regardless of movement in the arm. For this bit of sensory information, the

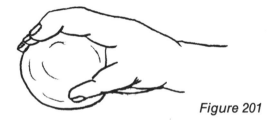

Figure 201

seven-month-old uses the mouth. Placing a toy in the mouth and holding it with the jaw as well as the hand, the child then moves the wrist and arm around (Figures 202-203). The child learns to maintain the grasp and can then wave the object around without accidentally dropping it. In other words, the grasp is isolated from other movements of the wrist and arm.

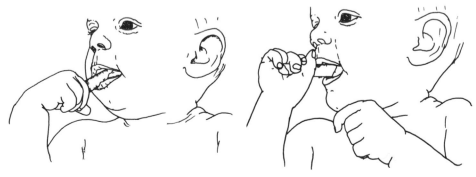

Figure 202   *Figure 203*

You can tug on the object playfully and the child will not let go. The seven-month-old feels powerful, grabbing anything interesting within reach. The child with a power grip can pull a tablecloth and completely dismantle a twelve-place dinner setting in less than seven seconds.

The process of development which allows the seven-month-old to create chaos in the home is the same process which allows the therapist to create success in treatment. The child experiences consistent hand contact with a variety of objects over a seven-month span. Remember this time span when you are waiting for your patients to make progress. It requires an infinite number of repetitions to establish a functional pattern in the hand.

Treatment strategies to shape the palmar grip

The following facilitation procedures can be utilized after you have expanded your patient's hand by inhibiting the abnormal tone. These procedures also can be used without inhibition since functional activity, in and of itself, may inhibit dysfunctional muscle tone. The techniques are more successful when the wrist is supported in a neutral position. It may help to support your patient's arm. These techniques can be used independently of each other. They are not listed in sequential order. Some are effective on spastic hands, while others work best on hypotonic or flaccid hands. What is important is that they do work. With many repetitions, they slowly improve the functional movement of the hand over a period of time.

It is important that you practice new techniques on a number of healthy hands first. This practice is your normal sensorimotor repetition. Without practice, it is difficult to choose the appropriate facilitation approach and know when it is working. Without feedback from your facilitation partner, it is difficult to learn to grade the amount of pressure needed during treatment.

As your patient attempts to grasp without palmar activity, the fingers may hyperextend and the grip will be weak (Figure 204). Palmar activity can be facilitated through the fingers of the therapist. Pressure onto the patient's mid palm with the pads of your index and middle fingers will facilitate palmar arches (Figure 205). You will place one or two of your fingers

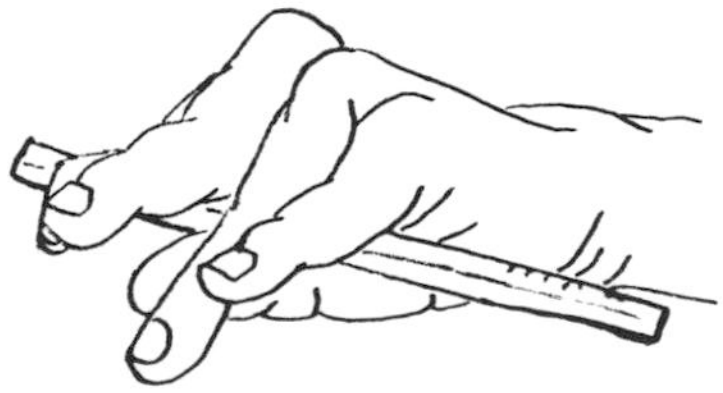

Figure 204

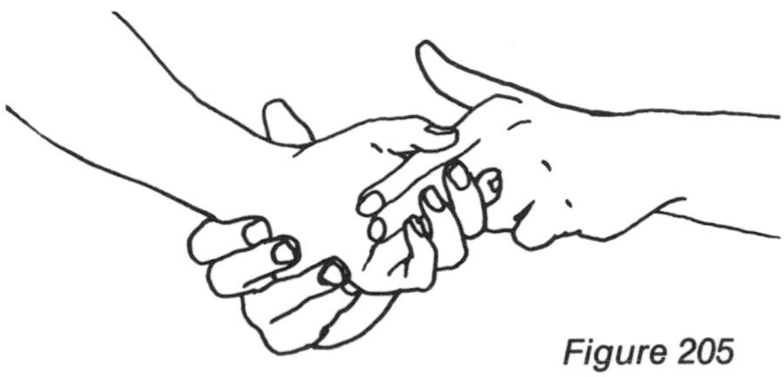

Figure 205

between the patient's thumb and index finger. But your patient will feel only your finger pads. If you traction slightly on the skin in the direction of the web space, the palm will activate. Palmar activity requires balanced movement between long finger flexors and extensors, along with intrinsic muscle activity. Maintaining your patient's wrist in neutral will ensure an equal amount of coactivation from both flexors and extensors. This procedure is especially productive when the patient is able to hold onto your fingers while you facilitate the arches (Figure 206). As you release your diagonal traction, the palmar activity will relax. The patient will develop prerequisite components for grasp and release on a very basic, kinesiological level. Facilitation of palmar activity will not create more spasticity because you can control the alignment of the wrist.

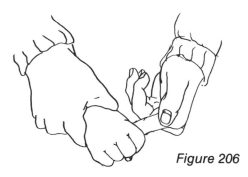

Figure 206

Because the hand is designed to shape itself around objects, you can mold your patient's hand around an object (Figure 207). Asking the patient to hold firmly, shape the fingers around the object. This will help develop the activity needed in the hand for gripping. A firm hold helps the patient feel the hand shape around the object. A firm hold will not create more abnormal tone, because you are controlling the alignment of the fingers.

Rolling the object into the palm is good sensory input for the hypotonic or flaccid hand (Figure 208). It is a distal-to-proximal facilitation for grasp.

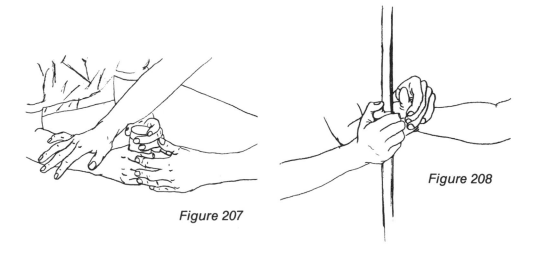

Figure 208

Figure 207

Facilitation of palmar and digital activity in the hypotonic hand can be accomplished with the gentle tugging of yarn or twine (Figure 209). As the digits become active, the palm will respond with activity. Another method to stimulate palmar activity is to shape the patient's fingers into an arch and then ask that the patient pull the hand away from you (Figure 210). In addition, you can place an object in the patient's hand and gently pull on it to create a slight resistance that will facilitate palmar arch activity (Figure 211).

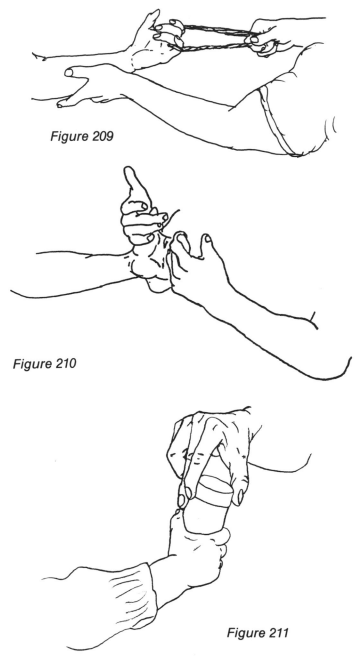

Figure 209

Figure 210

Figure 211

Arches in the hypotonic or flaccid hand can be activated by tapping the hand on the patient's knee, tapping the palm with a small ball, or tapping the palm with your finger pads (Figure 212). Tapping is used when there

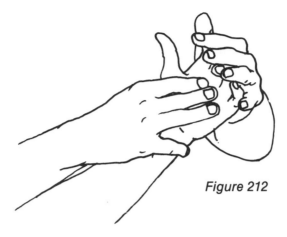

Figure 212

is apparent or real weakness of specific muscle groups or general hypotonia. It is not used with hypertonicity. Tapping produces an increase in tone and contractibility of muscles due to recruitment of central nervous system impulses. It often takes a series of taps before a response in the hand can be noticed. Each tap should be quickly followed by another. It is the repetition that builds the tone and enables the patient to hold the palmar activity long enough for you to place an object in the hand.

When any of the above procedures are used to stimulate a symmetrical grip, release should be facilitated as well. Initially, give your patient time to relax the grip sufficiently to allow you to roll the object out of the hand (Figure 213) or pull it easily from the hand.

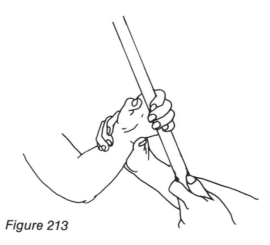

Figure 213

RELEASE

I have learned the developmental sequence of release from Rhoda Erhardt. Strategies to facilitate the component parts of active and controlled release come from analyzing her wonderful assessment scale (Erhardt 1982).

The development of release and its implications for treatment

Release develops off a point of stability, beginning with the mutual fingering in midline at four months of age. The child between five and six months of age learns to transfer from one hand to another. The infant starts with the object in hand #1, and places the object into hand #2. Hand #1 then releases off the stability provided by hand #1. Until the child develops this sensorimotor system, hand #2 will pull the object out of hand #1. Having the patient release with one hand stabilized against the other will facilitate a component part of hand-to-hand transfer (Figure 214).

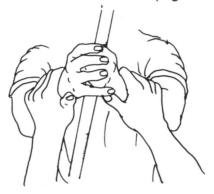

Figure 214

Children seem to use a similar sensorimotor procedure when they first hand an object to an adult. When the five-month-old offers a toy to an adult, the child does not immediately release it. In the past, I told audiences that the child was experimenting with social power. Everyone diligently enscribed this "fact." I hope you'll accept my apology today. The child cannot release the object to the adult until the stability provided by the adult's grasp is felt. Having the patient release an object while you are stabilizing it in space (Figure 215) will help develop this component part of a mature release. It is important to inhibit retraction of the arm and wait for the response to your facilitation. It often takes the patient time to use a new movement pattern.

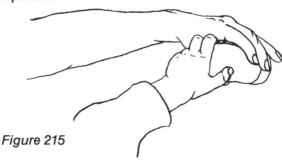

Figure 215

The seven-month-old can release an object on a highchair tray, the tray being the stable surface. But that same child, a moment later, cannot release an object in space. The seven-month-old does not have sufficient internal, dynamic stability to voluntarily open the hand to drop the toy in space. Releasing an object with the therapist stabilizing it against the surface will prepare the patient for release in space (Figure 216).

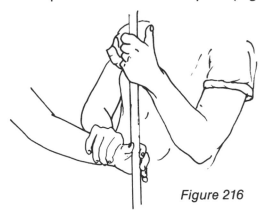

Figure 216

Patients with neurological deficits find other methods of releasing objects. They use wrist flexion which mechanically extends the fingers. They fling the object. They pull the object out of their hand. They abduct their humerus and straighten the elbow to synergistically extend the fingers. All of these methods work, but they limit the voluntary placement and control of the release. They do not allow the patient enough options for function.

Summary

Treatment strategies designed to help patients develop a mature, functional grasp and release take time and repetition. You are helping them make the most efficient adaptations to their dysfunctional tone. Splinting is a helpful way to maintain joint alignment outside of therapy (see Appendix A). Another option—inhibitory casting—can help you to reduce marked spasticity, increase range of motion, and improve joint alignment (see Appendix B). Inhibitory casting can be followed by a maintenance splinting program as well.

Once your patient develops a basic grip and can relax the grip adequately to roll the object out, you can begin to stimulate more mature hand patterns. The following chapter will focus on simple and complex movement blends in the hand.

References

Barnes, J. 1986. Myofascial Release I Seminar. Chicago, IL.

Erhardt, R. 1982. *Developmental hand dysfunction theory assessment treatment.* Laurel, MD: Ramsco Publishing Company.

Kapandji, I. 1982. Upper limb. In *The physiology of the joints,* Vol. I. New York: Churchill Livingstone.

Tubiana, R., J. Thomine, and E. Mackin. 1984. *Examination of the hand and upper limb.* Philadelphia: W.B. Saunders Company.

CHAPTER 6

Digital Manipulation

Introduction

Grasp and release are the least complex distal movement patterns. All digits move together or move apart in unison with basic patterns of flexion and extension. Both pinch and the dynamic tripod, seen in the pencil grip, utilize simple flexion and extension control. However, mastering buttons, zippers, shoelaces, scissors, and the variety of tools of our current technology demands more complex movement blends.

Fine motor blends are complex patterns of movement that utilize a combination of simple patterns, sequentially and concurrently, to perform a simple task. They involve the thumb's ability to move independent of the fingers, as in in-hand manipulation or the digital and wrist movement blends utilized in handwriting. Further, they may entail digital and palmar grip blends used with scissors and shoelaces. This chapter will provide you with an understanding of the hand's capacity for complex function. It will encourage methods of creative intervention that will ultimately lead your patient to a maximum level of autonomy.

Radial-Digital Grasp

Once your patient has established a power grip, encourage control of the digits. Gradually move an object away from the patient's palm toward the digits. Facilitate a digital grasp by your choice of placement and orientation of the object in the hand (Figure 217). This radial-digital grasp grips the object with an opposed thumb and fingertips (Erhard 1982). There is a

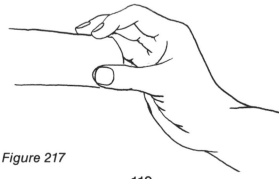

Figure 217

119

visible space within the palm. Once the eight-month-old has experienced this grasp with the wrist in a neutral position (Figure 218), this pattern will continue to be used, with the child varying the wrist position according to the spatial field (Figure 219). The radial-digital grasp relies on well-developed palmar arches.

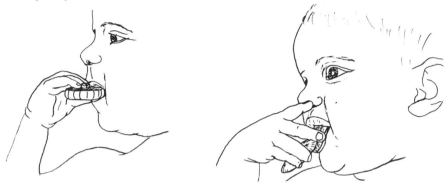

Figure 218   Figure 219

Three-Jawed Chuck

Specialized movement patterns in the ulnar and radial side of the hand are utilized for grasp of small objects as well as pointing. Interestingly, self-feeding provides valuable sensory information for this process (Figure 220). In addition, the eight- to ten-month-old child learns to isolate the digits on the radial side of the hand by holding a toy during quadruped movement (Figure 221). This sensorimotor experience of taking weight over the medial border of the hand concurrently with grasp helps establish the three-jaw chuck (Figure 222). Facilitation of radial and ulnar specialization is key to establishing efficient digital control. You can support the ulnar digits in the palm as you hand the patient an object.

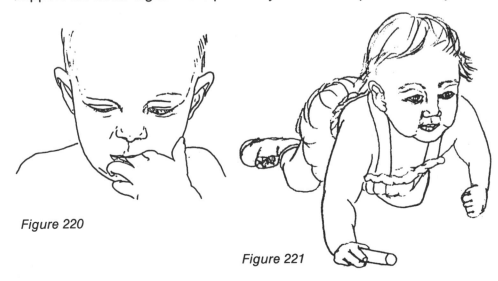

Figure 220

Figure 221

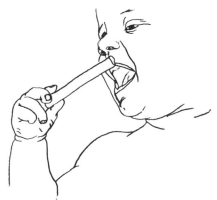

Figure 222

Pinch

As the child picks up smaller and smaller objects, one finger will slip away and the child will discover the pinch (Figure 223). Typically the middle finger moves toward the palm to act as a stabilizer. However, the hand that exhibits inadequate palm and wrist stability or limited thumb mobility will consistently use the middle finger rather than the index finger for pinch (Figure 224). A middle finger pinch, in and of itself, is not abnormal. In fact, it is used voluntarily when additional power is needed, but the normal hand is not obliged to use it. Because the index finger is needed for complex digital patterns, adapted hand patterns should be assessed and treated.

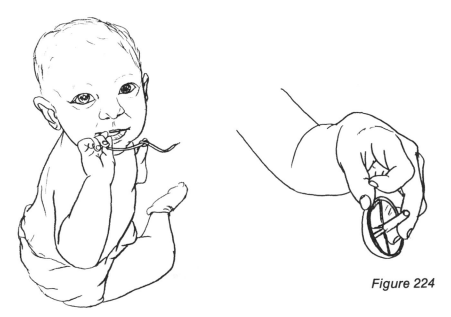

Figure 224

Figure 223

Pinch develops slowly off a stable surface and through successive approximation. It progresses from a crude attempt to capture the tiny object between the index and middle fingers at six months, to a lateral key-hold pinch at eight months (Figure 225) as well as a delicate fingertip pinch at twelve months (Figure 226) (Erhardt 1982). In treatment, your patient can work off the stability of a supporting surface to maintain the alignment of the wrist (Figure 227). In addition, your patient can begin to work off the support of your hand. Stabilizing the wrist as well as the base of the thumb will facilitate a working relationship between the thumb and index finger (Figure 228). A gentle tug on the object will facilitate strength and endurance in the pinch. Over time, the patient will develop the internal stability needed for simple digital control in space. Furthermore, your patient will use this internal stability for more complicated patterns.

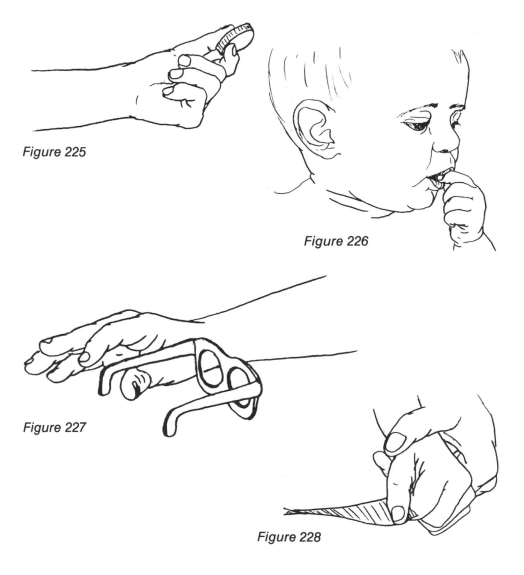

Figure 225

Figure 226

Figure 227

Figure 228

Reciprocal Patterns of Movement

Reciprocal patterns of movement reflect the thumb's ability to move independently of the fingers (Elliot and Connolly 1984). The digits involved in the function utilize dissimilar movements. For example, when winding a watch or a toy, the digits combine adduction of the thumb with flexion of the index finger (Figure 229). The reverse muscle actions are used to unwind. When this movement blend is absent, the patient will use whole-arm movements for winding and unwinding (Figure 230).

When screwing a lid onto a jar, the digits move in an ulnar direction while the thumb moves toward extension (Figure 231). When your patient cannot combine these components, a palmar grasp will be used to hold the lid, and whole-arm movements will be utilized either to replace or remove the lid. Again, inhibit the whole-arm movements and encourage your patient to find another way to complete the task. Your inhibition of whole-arm movements during the activity, in and of itself, will stimulate blended patterns.

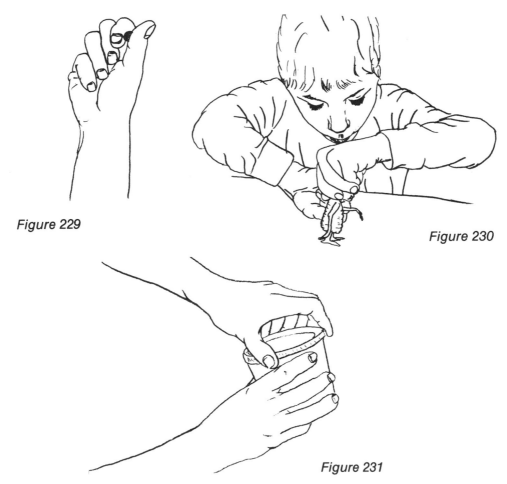

Figure 229

Figure 230

Figure 231

Sequential Patterns of Movement

An example of movement blends used sequentially is the rotation of a pencil in-hand for erasing (Figures 232-233). Patients who lack the components or the experience needed for motor sequencing will pronate the forearm to erase or transfer the pencil to the other hand (Figure 234). Inhibit their use of the second hand and encourage them to rotate the pencil in-hand, in any way that they are capable.

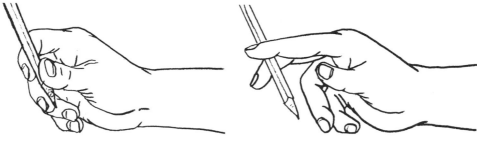

Figure 232   *Figure 233*

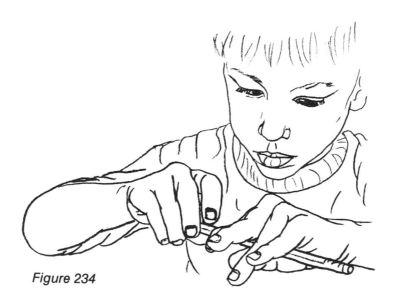

Figure 234

Sequencing is used for in-hand manipulation as well. Place an object in your patient's palm and ask the patient to turn it over, without using the second hand. Observe the blending and sequencing that occur during these attempts (Figures 235-238) Simple and reciprocal patterns of movement used in a sequence, bimanually, allow your patient success with buttons and jacket zippers, along with computer keyboards.

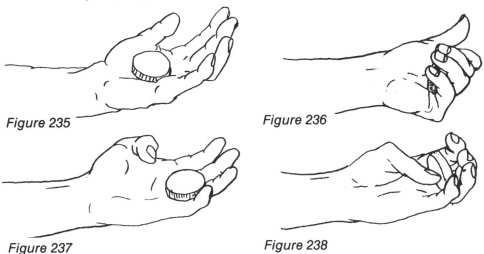

Figure 235

Figure 236

Figure 237

Figure 238

Writing and drawing require a different set of sequential movements. We know the dynamic tripod provides an efficient grip for writing tools (Figure 239). However, the ability to transfer information from thought to paper has less to do with the method of prehension and more to do with the ability

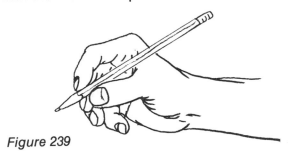

Figure 239

to combine and sequence digit and wrist movements. This is a blend of intrinsic and extrinsic muscle activity. Specifically, the flexion and extension movements of the digits produce the vertical excursion of the line. Lateral wrist movements produce the horizontal excursion of the line. Once this interplay is established, it is further integrated into the fluid ability to draw and write.

When the patient cannot combine digit and wrist movements, whole-arm movements will be substituted. Unfortunately, generating movement from the shoulder for writing is not efficient. It will require significant voluntary effort to grade the excursion of the line as well as pressure of the tool on the paper. In fact, the patient often attempts to stabilize off the tool by leaning it onto the paper.

Support your patient's forearm on the writing surface to discourage whole-arm movements. Gentle compression of the radius and ulna will provide additional stability. Allow the forearm to slide on the surface in response to the horizontal writing movements. As the patient learns to move wrist and digits sequentially, the motor components for writing will improve and specific perceptual dysfunction will be easier to identify. Carryover can be managed with the patient supporting the forearm while writing. To avoid slippage, the paper is held in a clipboard with nonskid backing.

Complex Patterns of Movement

When we firmly stabilize an object in the hand and concurrently manipulate it, we are combining precision with power. Shoe tying is a good example of this type of pattern in a matured form (Figures 240-241). The pattern is consistently refined for work-related or diversionally directed skills used thoughout life.

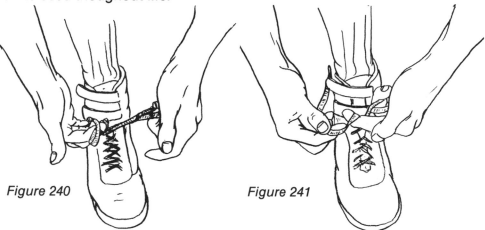

Figure 240   Figure 241

I usually begin by introducing simple parts of this complex pattern. The toothpaste pump is a useful tool to introduce the combination of stability with mobility (Figure 242). The fingers and palm stabilize the base while the thumb and palm mobilize the pump. This may be the reason Elliot and Connolly (1984) describe this pattern as "palmar combinations." Removing a pen cap with one hand will stimulate this pattern as well (Figure 243).

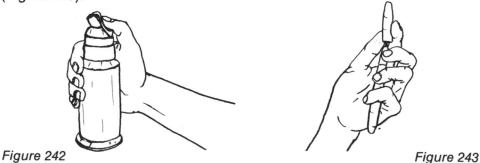

Figure 242   Figure 243

Both of these activities are component parts of scissor use (Figure 244). The digits stabilize the object, the thumb is the mover, and the wrist alters the orientation of the hand to the paper. To further complicate this process,

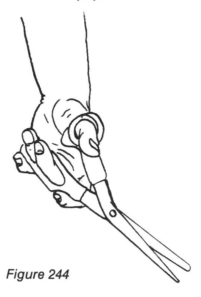

Figure 244

a second hand is used to hold the paper with the wrist altering the orientation of the paper in space. As these skills mature, they will become a complex, fluid interaction between two hands. When patients lack these complex movements, they learn to depend on the loop scissors.

I start my patient with the dressmaker's approach to cutting. The paper is held flat and the orientation of the scissors is altered by sliding and rotating it on the working surface. When treating the young at heart, I use the squirt gun. It requires a palmar combination utilizing the index finger as the mover. However, aiming at a target encourages the eyes to visualize ahead of the hand, an important component of cutting.

Mastering these complex patterns of movement offers your patient hope for autonomy in a world filled with safety caps, complicated clasps, protective seals, and remote controls.

References

Elliot, J., and K. Connolly. 1984. A classification of manipulative hand movements. *Developmental Medicine and Child Neurology* 26:283-296.

Erhardt, R. 1982. *Developmental hand dysfunction theory assessment treatment.* Laurel, MD: Ramsco Publishing Company.

Appendixes

Current Trends in Upper-Extremity Splinting

Susan G. Hill, O.T.R.

Introduction

Orthoses for the hands—often referred to as splints—are devices fitted to the arm which position or immobilize the hand and wrist for the purpose of relieving pain, preventing or correcting deformities, and substituting for loss of motor power (Trombly 1983; Malick 1980). The general intent of all splint designs is to maximize hand function for the individual (Fess, Gettle, and Strickland 1981). In some cases splints can be used as an aid in evaluating a patient's rehabilitation potential prior to surgical intervention (Hunter et al. 1983).

The orthoses discussed in this paper represent current trends in upper-extremity splinting. It is recommended that the reader refer to the references listed at the end of Appendix A for information on splints traditionally employed in the treatment of neurologically impaired patients.

Types of Splint

Three classifications of splints will be discussed in this paper. Static orthoses have no moving parts and serve to immobilize or "rest" the intended joints. Semidynamic orthoses also have no extrinsic moving parts but position joints so that the extremity can optimize its own available movement. The weight-bearing splint will be included in this group since it allows active transitional movement patterns. Dynamic orthoses employ moving parts (such as rubber bands, tension wires, springs, or elastic-like materials) to help the hand correct or compensate for muscle imbalance, increase range of motion, and improve joint alignment. The terms high and low profile, often used to describe dynamic splints, refer to the height of the traction device above the segment being mobilized (Hunter et al. 1983).

There are a number of commercially available "prefabricated" hand orthoses. However, these may not consistently fit well due to the number of anatomic and pathologic differences between patients (Cannon 1985; Johnstone 1978). For this reason the therapist is advised to design a specific splint pattern for each patient.

The materials used to construct hand orthotics will vary, depending on the individual needs of the patient and the therapist's preference of materials. Low-temperature thermoplastics (LTT) are commonly used to fabricate hand orthoses due to their relative low cost, ease in use, and lightweight and attractive appearance.

The Controversy Surrounding Splinting Practices

Over the past 100 years, there has been a tremendous discrepancy in splinting practices, just as there have been differences in treatment approach for the neurologically impaired. Neuhaus and colleagues, in *A survey of rationales for and against hand splinting in hemiplegia* (1981), found that therapists with a longer clinical experience using orthosis had a greater tendency to splint than those with less experience. Yet within this group, there were conflicting opinions concerning when splints are indicated.

In investigating the controversy, the authors identified two different approaches to treatment for hemiplegia which greatly impacted on current splinting practices. The biomechanical approach, documented primarily between the early 1900s through the 1950s, emphasized the prevention or correction of deformity by mechanical application of splints, towel rolls, and sand bags used in conjunction with passive range of motion (PROM). The neurophysiological treatment approach which emerged in the 1950s concentrated on the use of movement and handling techniques to reduce spasticity. Although it too emphasized prevention of deformity, traditional splints were either not included or were opposed.

Bobath, Brunnstrom, and Rood were among the first therapists to suggest viable alternatives to traditional biomechanical approaches such as splinting (Bobath 1971; Brunnstrom 1956). Rood, in particular, cautioned that splints may actually stimulate spasticity "by activating sensory stimuli of touch, pressure, and stretch, which result in undesirable contraction of muscle" (1954).

To date, there is little research, either qualitative or quantitative, which conclusively supports or disputes use of any one approach to splinting. There is a great variance in the recommended wearing times, the types of materials used, and where the splint material should be placed on the upper extremity. For example, Brennon (1959) reported decreased spasticity in fourteen hemiplegic patients who wore splints almost constantly for three to five months, whereas McPherson (1981) reported decreased spasticity in subjects who wore splints for a maximum of two hours daily for four weeks. Others, such as Kaplan (1982), investigated the use of different splint materials. He designed a dorsal-based splint made of plaster and fiberglass which was lined with textured material for stimulation of the extensor muscles. Blashy and Fuchs (1959) developed an orthokinetic cuff splint which combined elastic and nonelastic materials. Jamison and Dayhoff (1980) reported success in the use of a hard hand-positioning device to decrease hypertonicity. Finally, a combination of the hard positioning device with the dynamic orthokinetic cuff was described by Farber and Huss (1974).

Mills (1984) conducted one of the few electromyographic (EMG) studies comparing splinted and nonsplinted conditions. This researcher reported a significant change in joint position, utilizing a bivalved circumferential splint. She explains that the range of motion is increased due to the muscle groups accommodating to the position of the splint rather than a change in EMG activity.

Dorsal versus Volar Placement

A number of researchers compared dorsal versus volar splint placement, again yielding a wide variety of results. It appears that differences in research design and methodology, lack of continuity between studies, and inadequate documentation to support the investigators' conclusions may account for the discrepancy between the studies. Charait (1968) reported that dorsal splinting was more effective in reducing spacticity. Zizlis (1964) reported decreased flexor activity in a hemiparetic adult who was changed from a dorsal-based, finger-adduction splint to a volar-based, finger-abduction splint. Doubilet and Polkow (1977) reported successful utilization of a hand-based finger-abduction splint for reducing spasticity. Finally, McPherson et al. (1980) compared use of a dorsal-based splint developed by Snook (1981) with a similar volar-based splint. McPherson's group found that both splints reduced hypertonus and that the age of the patient had a significant effect on tonal reduction. The younger the client, the more significant the reduction in hypertonus. In light of the findings of McPherson et al. (1980), it is reasonable to assume the plausibility of using splints for treating hypertonicity in children with the same or similar disabilities as adults, such as cerebral palsy (Gesell and Amatruda 1949; Bobath and Bobath 1964, 1975; Erhardt 1982).

Pediatric Splinting

Whereas there is little documentation supporting splinting practices in adults, there is even less research published that demonstrates the efficacy of splinting children with spasticity. Certainly the condition of cerebral palsy poses inherent research problems from a scientific, quantitative perspective. There is a lack of uniform means for measuring spasticity, isolation of the variables affecting tone, and the mixture of tones presented by some cerebral palsied patients. The bulk of the literature is descriptive in nature. One study by Exner and Bonder (1983) compared use of the MacKinnon splint, the orthokinetic cuff, and the short opponens thumb splint in children. They suggested that the MacKinnon splint was more likely associated with improvement in bilateral hand use and grasp skill.

The Proper Perspective

Despite the number of studies reporting gains in range of motion and reduction of hypertonus, few studies report gains in hand function. This observation may lead the reader to consider that orthoses, like any other therapeutic intervention for the hand, cannot be used in isolation (Grossman, Sahrmann, and Rose 1982). Rather, splints are used as an adjunct to other therapeutic techniques to help increase the functional use of the involved limb.

Principles of Splinting

Numerous low-temperature thermoplastics (LTT) are manufactured for use in hand orthotics, each with individual advantages and disadvantages. Table 1 (pages 136-137) describes and compares the characteristics of many currently available LTTs. I recommend that you become familiar with and adept in using one or two types of materials.

Before recommending a splint, identify your therapeutic goals. Splinting can increase function by providing support and protection for weak muscles as well as diseased and painful joints. It offers proximal stability for distal control and can help the patient efficiently substitute for loss of muscle function. Maintaining a comfortable position in the hand can reduce edema, prevent or decrease deformities, and ease the problems with skin care.

PRECAUTIONS RELATIVE TO SPLINT DESIGN

As you design the splint, use your favorite anatomy book and consider the anatomical structure of the hand. For example, the transverse and longitudinal arches of the hand should be supported to preserve proper joint alignment and provide comfort.

For example, the distal palmar crease should be clear of obstruction to allow for full flexion of the MP joints. The thenar and finger creases remain clear so that thumb abduction and opposition can take place. Pressure is avoided over body prominences of the hand and wrist. The most common problem sites include the MP joints, ulnar and radial styloid processes, and the area surrounding the pisiform. Compression of the superficial branch of the radial nerve may occur if a forearm-based splint extends beyond the mid-lateral aspect of the forearm around the dorsum of the thumb.

Avoid over-splinting. It is important to stabilize the bone proximal to the joint being mobilized. However, it is equally important not to unnecessarily immobilize joints. A careful analysis of your goals and assessment of the patient will help with the splint's design.

Lateral stress to joints should be avoided. Such stress may cause unequal stretching of the collateral ligaments. For example, an incorrect angle of pull applied to a finger during dynamic splinting will cause the finger to drift out of alignment. The ulnar collateral ligament of the thumb may be particularly vulnerable to ligamentous stress during construction of a thumb-abduction splint. Do not overstretch the web space as you position the thumb in radial or palmar abduction. Regarding ligamentus shortening, it is important to avoid secondary shortening of laxed collateral ligaments that may occur when the MP joints are immobilized over a long period of time. Range-of-motion exercises will help prevent joint immobility secondary to splinting.

In cases of edema, increase the area of coverage and use wide straps to minimize further swelling. The splint can be removed every hour for nonresistive range-of-motion exercises, allowing the muscles to pump fluid back into the system. When a traction device is applied, use a low amount of traction over a long period of time. Two hours would be advised in order to produce a viscoelastic response and prevent inflammation. Elasticized bandage wrap or stockinette, along with intermittent elevation, can help control edema.

PRECAUTIONS RELATIVE TO FABRICATION

Kinesiology and biomechanics are important considerations during fabrication. For example, as the fingers and thumb move through an arc of motion during hand use, the anatomical configurations of the hand change. The splint is designed to accommodate the anticipated changes in the arches and bony prominences. Otherwise, motion may be inhibited and pressure areas can occur. Articulated splints, such as the orthokinetic wrist splint, align the rotational axis of the splint with the anatomic axis of the wrist joint. This will allow unhampered movement at the joint.

By increasing the area of force application, you will decrease the pressure to the cutaneous surface and underlying soft tissue. Consequently, wider splints and straps will be more comfortable than short, narrow ones. Splints which cross the wrist should extend two-thirds the length and one-half the width of the forearm so the weight of the hand will be more evenly distributed through the forearm trough. In addition, the edges of the splint should be rolled to reduce uncomfortable pressure input. Continuous, uniform pressure over a bony prominence will reduce potential soft tissue damage.

Dynamic traction should be applied at a 90-degree angle to the segment being mobilized. This will maximize the force potential of the traction device without producing an undesirable traction or compression force on the articular surface of the involved joint. In most situations, the line of pull

TABLE 1

Comparison of Low-Temperature Thermoplastic (LTT) Splinting Materials

Trade Name	Recommended Heat Source and Temperature	Working Characteristics	Positive Features
Aquaplast	Wet heat, using an Aquaplast Frypan Guard to prevent material from sticking to pan At 140° F, becomes elastic; working temperature is 160–180° F	Becomes transparent and sticky when soft; therapist must use hand lotion or keep hands wet during splint fabrication Moderate rigidity when hard Material shrinks as it cools; therapist may need to enlarge openings to compensate for this Careful handling is required to avoid accidental bonding Recommended for use by more experienced splinter	Clings to extremity during molding; highly conforming Requires no preparation to self-bond Returns to original shape when reheated Placement of splint aided by transparency Manufacturer reports material cannot be overheated (at 160–180° F) Color change indicates softening and hardening
Aquaplast-T	Similar to Aquaplast	Becomes transparent but slightly cloudy when soft Nonsticky surface To bond, use solvent, abrasion, and/or spot heat until shiny	Has advantages similar to Aquaplast Does not cling as well as Aquaplast yet easier to handle Highly conforming
Polyform Kay Splint	Wet heat These materials remain firm to 150° F, then become moldable Range: 150–160° F	Lack of rubber content makes the material nonelastic and very pliable when soft Pliability is adjustable with water temperature Working time is 3–5 minutes If you can position your client in a gravity-assisted position, the material will practically mold itself Edges finish easily by dipping in hot water and smoothing	Excellent rigidity and conformity Bonds well with surface preparation and heat to both surfaces Material has no shelf life

Material	Heat	Properties	Comments
Ultra Form	Wet heat Range: 140-160° F	Similar to Polyform and Kay Splint Working time is 3-4 minutes Bonds with solvent and heat to one surface	Excellent conformity Resists fingerprints
Kay Splint (Isoprene) Polyflex II	Wet heat Softens at 150° F Range: 150-160° F	Similar to Polyform and Kay Splint except has a slight resistance to stretch when molding and less rigid when hard Controlled stretch (resilient) Bonds well with solvent	Greater temperature tolerance Material is highly conforming yet has controlled stretch Rapid cooling of material is better tolerated by patients with heat sensitivity Good material of choice when fabricating splints requiring circumferential design, as it does not stress fracture from repetitive opening and closing
Ultra Form 294	Wet heat Range: 160-170° F	Similar to Kay Splint (Isoprene) and Polyflex II, possibly more stretch resistant Working time: 4-6 minutes Bonds with solvent and heat one surface	
Ezeform Orthoplast San-Splint	Wet heat preferred Range: 160-170° F for Ezeform and Orthoplast; 175° F for San-Splint Softens slowly as temperature increases Orthoplast and San-Splint can be heated in a dry electric pan or oven, using a cookie sheet to prevent sticking	Orthoplast and San-Splint have high rubber content, making material elastic and least contouring of plastics previously mentioned Ezeform has no rubber, rather is plastic which yields greater conformability then Orthoplast or San-Splint, yet has a controlled stretch similar to the rubber-based materials Works well under wide temperature range Working time is 4-6 minutes; cools in 8-10 minutes. Time for hardening can be accelerated with cold water or cold spray Materials will bond to themselves if overlapped, but bonds best after using solvent to remove surface oils	Orthoplast and San-Splint are semirigid when hard; Ezeform has excellent rigidity Good material of choice when fabricating splints which require less contouring and quick cooling, yet longer time to harden., such as splints which inhibit spasticity Translucent to x-rays

should be perpendicular to the joint axis to prevent stress of collateral ligaments (Figure 245). Finger flexion is the exception to this rule, since the line of pull is directed toward the scaphoid bone in the carpus.

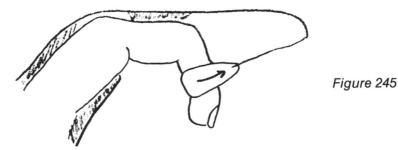

Figure 245

A properly fitted splint does not create friction. Improper fit of the splint, poor joint alignment, and inefficient fastening devices may cause skin irritation and eventual breakdown. Generally speaking, if the splint is worn for one-half hour and causes a red pressure sore on the skin, the redness should disappear within 15 to 20 minutes after splint removal. If it does not, correct the frictional problem.

In some cases, moleskin on the splint or gauze placed between two cutaneous surfaces can help eliminate friction. Padding can be used with certain restrictions. As a general rule, avoid padding as a way to compensate for improper fit of the splint. Do not add padding over a bony prominence with prior flaring out of the splint material. Otherwise, the padding will actually increase the pressure. In cases of spasticity, avoid padding the volar-based arm splint, as it theoretically may be facilitatory to the flexor musculature.

MONITORING THE SPLINTED PATIENT

It is important to establish a wearing schedule prior to dispensing the splint for use outside the clinic. The length of wearing time is balanced with a period of splint removal for the purpose of skin inspection, maintenance of hygiene, and exercise. For splints designed to correct deformities, the initial wearing period may be 5 to 10 minutes, whereas a purely supportive splint can be worn for approximately 30 minutes initially. The wearing time is gradually increased as tolerated.

Spastic extremities are splinted in a submaximal range and removed frequently for exercise. This procedure is recommended to avoid the tendency of spasticity to travel to an unsplinted joint. It may be preferable to splint the patient with spasticity during sleep where dysfunctional muscle tone will not have the opportunity to work against the alignment of the hand in the splint.

Before you send the splint home with the patient, evaluate it for comfort, fit, and function (Table 2). Consider the cooperation and interest of the patient and family members, by developing a realistic splint wearing and exercise schedule.

TABLE 2
Checklist for Hand Splints

YES	NO	

FIT

1. Is the splint positioned correctly?
2. Does the splint needlessly immobilize a joint?
3. Is available ROM permitted at wrist, thumb and finger, MP and IP joints as desired? Does the palmar bar fit proximal to the distal palmar crease so that it does not interfere with MP flexion?
4. Are all bony prominences free from pressure?
5. Is the forearm trough two-thirds the length and one-half the width of the forearm? Does it conform to the contour of the arm?
6. Are all splint joints in alignment with their corresponding anatomical joints?
7. Are the natural arches of the hand preserved?
8. After wearing the splint for one-half hour, does the individual have reddened areas? Do these disappear within 15 to 20 minutes after splint removal?
9. If elastics are used, do they have the correct perpendicular pull?
10. Is the splint adjusted periodically to keep up with changes in muscle tone and ROM?
11. In cases of spasticity, is the joint splinted in submaximum range and then gradually increased to a position of function (15 to 30° of dorsiflexion)?

COMFORT

1. Is the splint comfortable? If not, can the fit be improved? Can the dynamic forces be adjusted?
2. Will added padding actually increase pressure? If padding was added, was adequate space allowed by spot-heating the LTT?
3. Are the inside edges and rivets smooth to prevent skin abrasions?
4. Can the patient tolerate the splint for the recommended wearing time without experiencing discomfort?
5. Is perspiration a problem? Can the material be ventilated? Can cotton stockinette be tolerated?

FUNCTION

1. Does the splint accomplish its intended purpose?
2. Is the splint cosmetically attractive?
3. Is the splint easy to apply and remove?
4. When relaxed, is the hand in as functional a position as passive joint range will permit?
5. Does the splint restrict forearm pronation, thereby interfering with effective prehension?
6. Is the splint designed to improve prehension? Do the index and middle finger pads have maximum contact with the thumb pad? Does this splint permit functional grasp of small and large objects?
7. Is release of objects adequate for function?
8. Is splint construction sturdy enough to support the wrist as the individual removes the fingers or thumb?
9. Has a realistic wearing schedule been established?
10. If the splint immobilizes one or more joints, is it removed periodically for ROM?
11. Can wearing of the splint be reduced as active movement improves?

Static Splints

Static orthosis have no moving parts and serve to immobilize or rest the intended joints.

SPASTICITY REDUCTION SPLINT

History and design rationale

Based on the work of Bobath (1971), Julie Hindenach Snook, OTR, developed this splint for the purpose of reducing tone in a hand dominated by flexor spasticity resulting from hemiplegia (secondary to a CVA) or brain damage. It was designed to maintain the hand in a reflex inhibitory posture (RIP) which includes wrist, fingers (IP joints), and thumb extension, as well as finger abduction. In addition, the splint was dorsally based to avoid the uncertain, yet possibly stimulatory, effect of a forearm trough on the volar aspect of the arm.

Indications

For children and adults with varying degrees of spasticity. It works best for individuals who have recently developed spasticity.

Materials and construction

Generally speaking, two persons are needed to fabricate the splint. One person positions the patient and the other molds the splint material. Snook has recommended using the RIP in the hand prior to fitting the splint. In cases of more severe spasticity, she recommended first reducing the tone at the shoulder using additional Bobath techniques. A pattern can be made by modifying a dorsal resting pan or a mitt-shaped splint pattern, increasing the width of the palmar finger pan with an extra "fold" of material allowed at the MP joints for reinforcement purposes. The designer has recommended use of a highly conforming low-temperature plastic which offers a moderate to high level of rigidity when it hardens.

Steps for fabrication (Figure 246)

1. Heat and mold the forearm trough up to the MP cut-out section. Position the wrist in approximately 30 degrees of extension, checking for proper wrist alignment before the material hardens.

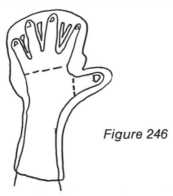

Figure 246

2. Heat and mold the finger pan. The pan is molded on a firm surface, not on the spastic extremity. Snook recommends molding the finger pan on the edge of a level surface such as a table top, so the pan would remain flat. However, you may mold the finger pan on a rounded surface such, as a mid-sized ball, so that the IP joints are positioned in slight flexion (Figure 247). This will help prevent hyperextension of MP and IP joints, which may occur during splint wearing as an "expression" of tight finger flexors. Build in a palmar arch as the material hardens. The dorsal portion of the splint is angled, at the cut section, to achieve a 45-degree flexion angle at the MP's joints.

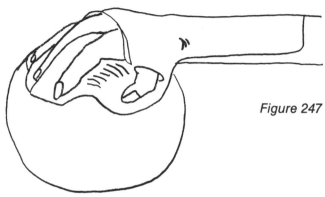

Figure 247

3. Apply the splint to the individual, marking and adding finger abductors. V-shaped separators are used between the index and middle as well as middle and ring fingers. A 1-shaped separator is used between the ring and little fingers.

4. Heat and mold the thumb trough so that the thumb is positioned in extension.

5. Round and smooth all edges. A strip of splint material can be added behind the thumb trough and across the finger pan to reinforce the splint.

6. The designer has recommended use of 2" strapping at the wrist and 1" strapping at the fingers, thumb, and forearm.

Correct fit
The degree of wrist extension may be varied from 30 degrees to neutral or slightly below as range of motion and comfort will permit. The MPs are flexed approximately 45 degrees. The fingers should be abducted and slightly flexed at the IP joints. Full index finger abduction and thumb extension and abduction are critical for control in the RIP. For ease of application, the splint is held upside down and parallel with the hand. Next the fingers and thumb are inserted into their respective openings. When the fingers and thumb are in place, the forearm trough can be flipped over so that it fits on the dorsum of the arm. The splint will fit "snugly," supporting the IP and MP joints.

Alternate fit

Fabricate the splint so it is volar based. Allow extra width in the resting pan section to form finger separators and thumb trough.

Precautions

1. Watch for boutonniere or swan neck deformities in the fingers during splint wearing.

2. This splint may work best for individuals who have recently developed spasticity as opposed to those who have developed severe spasticity and contractures.

3. The arm and hand must be observed frequently for pressure areas.

4. Caretakers are often confused by the application of the splint and may try to put it on "upside down." Additional demonstrations or a photograph of the proper fit may be helpful.

Wearing time

An intermittent wearing schedule (such as two hours on, one hour off) should be maintained; otherwise, after an extended period of time, tone may gradually increase. Therapeutic exercise can take place during the time-off periods. Nighttime wearing is recommended, as tolerated. If tone is not reduced within a two-week period, consider utilizing other means for reducing spasticity.

FINGER ABDUCTION SPLINT

History and design rationale

Originally fabricated from a strip of foam (3" x 2" x 1½") that was perforated with four holes, this spasticity inhibition splint was designed to duplicate a reflex-inhibiting posture of Bobath. Theoretically, by maintaining the MP joints of the fingers in abduction, the splint would simultaneously inhibit flexion while aiding extension.

Due to the poor durability of the foam material, Doubilet and Polkow (1977) redesigned the splint using thermoplastics. LTTs which are semirigid when hard were the materials found to be suitable for ease of fabrication, time, and expense. Doubilet and colleague reported moderate reduction in spasticity in fifteen patients, two to six months post cerebral vascular accident (CVA), who exhibited moderate to severe spasticity of the fingers and wrist. The splint was worn for one week, removed during therapy, an hour at each meal time, and at night. No attempt was made to describe how spasticity was measured or to isolate the effect of the splint versus the effect of other therapeutic techniques.

Indications

1. For individuals with moderate to severe spasticity of the fingers and wrist

2. Extremity may be edematous and have decreased joint range

Materials and construction (Figure 248)
1. Measure and cut out a piece of LTT approximately the length of the fingers and the width of the patient's hand with the thumb abducted. The size of the material will vary according to the size of the patient's hand. For a small adult this may be 8" x 3".

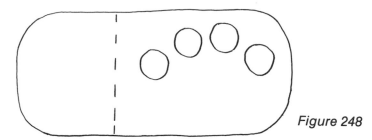

Figure 248

2. Place fingers in a comfortable amount of abduction, and mark the finger position on the splint material.

3. Heat the material slightly and, using a leather punch, make four holes for the fingers. Arrange the holes in a slight arch, following the natural shape of the hand.

4. Reheat the LTT. Widen the holes prior to fitting the material on the patient's hand.

5. Fit the splint on the patient between the PIP and DIP joints with the wrist positioned in neutral. The ulnar side of the splint should be pulled downward toward the ulnar side of the hand for a better fit. The lower edge can be pulled outward to form a base for positioning on a table top.

6. After the material is completely hardened, heat only the thumb section of the material until pliable.

7. Fit the splint back on the patient. While holding the thumb in a comfortable degree of extension, mold the material to form a lateral C-bar.

8. When the material is sufficiently hardened, reheat and trim the C-bar to conform to the size of the patient's thumb. Round and smooth all other edges.

Correct fit
Fingers should be placed in enough abduction so that the splint can be tolerated for an extended period of wearing time without discomfort. The opening for the fingers should be maintained between the PIP and DIP joints of the fingers. A strap can be added to secure the splint in position, especially for use during ambulation.

Alternate fit
The thumb can be positioned in abduction, molding the splint material around the thumb from the medial to the lateral side.

Precautions
When fitting the splint on the fingers, avoid ulnar or radial deviation at the MP joints. When using a highly elastic LTT, allow extra widening of the finger holes to accommodate for shrinking of material as it cools and hardens. Otherwise the splint may cause irritation and pressure on the fingers. Once spasticity has been reduced, the splint should be discontinued and other therapy techniques emphasized.

PNEUMATIC SPLINTS

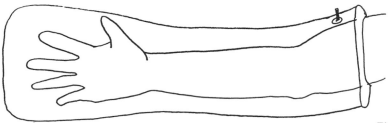

Figure 249

History and design rationale
In 1977, Boch and Evans published an article which introduced an inflatable splint for the spastic hand. This consisted of three pieces of canvas sewn into a "glove." It was inflated by means of a pediatric blood pressure cuff, maintained in a pocket underneath the palm. As the "glove cuff" was inflated, extension of the hand at both the MP and PIP joints was achieved. The designers cited one case in which the pneumatic splint helped reduce contractures in a 19-year-old head-injury patient who was displaying decorticate spasticity. They reported that after two weeks of application, the contracture in both MPs and PIPs were reduced sufficiently so that a fixed or static splint could be applied. No other publications were found describing the use of this splint.

The pneumatic splints currently available on the market were originally designed for emergency immobilization of an injured limb. Pneumatic splints are commonly referred to as air bag splints. They have been successfully used in the treatment of fractures, lower extremity amputations and edematous extremities secondary to trauma, vascular disturbances, or prolonged statis.

The air bag splint has a number of applications for the treatment of neurologically impaired individuals. In the case of flaccid hemiplegia, the splint can be used to reduce edema by mobilizing tissue fluid into the general circulation. It provides uniform pressure over the edematous area which is easily observable through the transparent material of the splint. By alternating use of the splint with range-of-motion and other therapeutic activities, joint mobility can be enhanced in the edematous and nonedematous "stiff" hand. Greenberg and Braun (1977) reported that, depending on the hand position in the splint, pressure exerted on the dorsal and volar surfaces of the hand can increase finger flexion or extension.

Further, the splint can reduce spasticity by maintaining the arm in the reflex-inhibiting pattern of external shoulder rotation, elbow, wrist, and finger extension with thumb abduction. The pneumatic cushioning of the inflated splint conforms to the shape of the limb and supports the arm in extension, allowing the therapist to concentrate on muscle re-education at the shoulder. Johnstone (1975) has recommended that movement re-education be conducted twice a day for 15 to 20 minutes with the splint on. This is followed by weight bearing through the extended arm with the splint off.

Indications
1. For individuals with flaccid hemiplegia or mild to moderate spasticity

2. For individuals who have stiff joints secondary to edema or muscle tightness

Materials and construction
The pneumatic splints are relatively inexpensive, lightweight, durable, and simple to clean. They are easy to apply with a full-length zipper and a self-closing inflation tube.

Correct fit
These splints are available in half- and full-arm, adult and child sizes. The therapist is advised to consult the manufacturer's guidelines for the correct fitting of the splint. The arm positioned in a reflex-inhibiting posture of external shoulder rotation, elbow, wrist, and finger extension, and thumb abduction is suggested in cases of spasticity.

Precautions
1. The individual may experience some discomfort due to perspiration. Using a layer of cotton stockinette between the extremity and the plastic will help relieve this.

2. The splints should not be worn overnight.

3. There is a risk that the inflation pressure of the splint can cause tissue necrosis. Monitor the skin for color and temperature, removing the splint if circulatory problems are observed.

4. In cases of spasticity, do not leave the splint on for more than 15 minutes. The heat generated by wearing the splint may actually increase hypertonus in the extremity.

Semidynamic Splints

Semidynamic orthoses have no extrinsic moving parts. However, they do position the hand and wrist so that the extremity can optimize its own movement.

THUMB LOOP

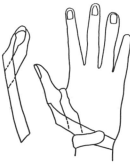

Figure 250

History and design rationale

It has been theorized that thumb extension with abduction can help inhibit abnormal tone in the hand and arm. Developed originally by Jan Utley, P.T., for the treatment of head-injured adults, the thumb loop splint is designed specifically to inhibit tone and to "normalize" hand function by facilitating wrist and thumb alignment. This is accomplished by the pull of the strapping material which rotates the metacarpal of the thumb into radial abduction while simultaneously pulling the wrist into an extended and radially deviated position. The hand not only gains a better position for prehension, manipulation, and release of objects but also gains the freedom of movement needed for bilateral motor coordination.

No literature has been published regarding the use of this splint. In a year-long study investigating the effects of splinting on children with spasticity (Hill 1985), I found that the thumb loop splint had an immediate effect on aligning the wrist and positioning the thumb in abduction. Compared with other splints in the study, it was the least restrictive, allowing the hand to grasp objects of different sizes. Additionally, it was quick and easy to fabricate and was tolerated well by the children in the study.

Indications

For any patient who has increased tone in the hand and arm secondary to an upper-motor neuron lesion

Materials

1. Use 1" cotton webbing or velcro loop material. I prefer using Duraval (Aquaplast Corp.) strapping for this splint due to its durability, smooth finished edge when cut, and its ability to adhere to velcro hook. Other therapists have reported successful use of Neoplush (Dricast Orthopaedics) for making this splint. The width of the material can be decreased for a small child.

2. Moleskin can be used with webbing or velcro loop to increase comfort and keep the cotton webbing strap from fraying where it has been cut.

3. Velcro hook and loop, approximately 1½″ of each.

Construction

1. With the hand held in neutral, hold the strap to the radial, dorsal side of the wrist. Bring the strap volar to dorsal through the web space so it wraps around the thumb and crosses over itself at the first metacarpophalangeal joint, forming a loop.

2. Mark and cut out concave strips from both sides of the strapping so that the thumb loop fits smoothly around the dorsal interossei and thenar eminence of the thumb. Add moleskin to the webbing as needed.

3. Reshape the thumb loop around the first metacarpal, securing the strap in place with self-adhesive velcro loop and hook. Adjust the angle of pull of the strapping so the thumb is in radial abduction.

4. Pull the other end of the strap dorsally at a slight angle so that it rests over the ulnar styloid process and continue wrapping it one time around the wrist. Cut it midway along the dorsal aspect of the wrist.

5. Secure this end of the strap in place with velcro hook on the underside of this end of the strap.

6. Sew all velcro strips onto the strapping. You may wish to sew the strapping at the point where it crosses to form the thumb loop as this will save time when fitting the thumb loop for subsequent use.

Correct fit

Leave ample time for fitting. The tension of the strap should be sufficient to pull the wrist into slight extension and radial deviation. Keep in mind that the anatomical structures of the hand and wrist change their relationships as the hand becomes more relaxed. The thumb loop may need adjustment one or two times each 45-minute treatment session. The strapping should provide sufficient support to the shaft of the first metacarpal without crossing over the thenar eminence.

Alternative method for fitting thumb loop

For those individuals who are unable to open their hand during wrist extension due to tight finger flexors, the strap can be wrapped differently to facilitate finger extension with the wrist in a more neutral position. This can be accomplished by starting the strap at the middle of the wrist, volar aspect. Bring the strap volar to dorsal through the web space so the strap fits smoothly around the thumb and crosses over itself. Secure it in place. Pull the other end of the strap toward the ulnar side of the hand and wrap it dorsal to volar to dorsal, one time over the ulnar styloid process. Complete as described above.

Deviation cuff modification

The thumb loop can be modified to be slightly more supportive by adding a deviation cuff made of low-temperature plastic (LTT). The pull of the strapping through the ulnar border piece serves to inhibit ulnar deviation. In addition, during weight bearing, it may facilitate relaxation of the hand such that the fingers abduct to meet the change in alignment of the other anatomical structures of the wrist and hand.

For maximum function and comfort, the deviation cuff must fit between the distal palmar transverse crease and the middle palmar crease. The edges should be slightly flared to prevent pressure areas.

I suggest fabricating the thumb loop portion of the splint first, temporarily securing the loop in place using self-adhesive velcro closures. The ulnar cuff is fabricated next. A 1″ slit is cut into the dorsal surface of the cuff, large enough for strapping to go through (Figure 251). The cuff is then secured to the thumb loop using a rivet made of either LTT or metal.

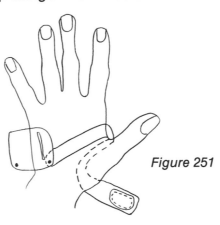

Figure 251

A second strap is riveted to the base of the deviation cuff on the volar side (Figure 252). This is drawn volar to dorsal under the first strap and through the opening in the cuff. It is then pulled back onto itself and fastened into place using velcro closures. The strapping can be contoured to fit into the opening as needed.

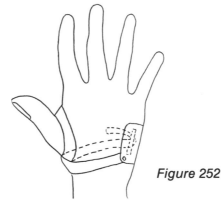

Figure 252

Once the deviation cuff is in place, the thumb loop can be readjusted to achieve the desired position of the thumb abduction and extension. The thumb loop and velcro closures are then sewn into place. The rivets must be flush with the interior surface of the deviation cuff and may be covered with moleskin.

Precautions

Hyperextension of the IP or MP joint of the thumb may occur during activity, if the individual has tight or contracted thumb adductors. This should be carefully monitored. This splint may be contraindicated in an individual with an extremely unstable thumb. In such cases, a thumb post or other more supportive splint may be indicated. Finally, watch that the strap of the thumb loop does not cross over the thenar eminence, as this may facilitate thumb adduction.

WEIGHT-BEARING HAND SPLINT

History and design rationale

Developed in 1981 by pediatric physical therapist Linda A. Lindholm, the splint is designed to duplicate the position that the upper extremity normally assumes in a weight-bearing situation (Lindholm 1985). It is felt that pressure exerted on the tendons of spastic muscles will have an inhibitory effect on these muscles.

Worn during neurodevelopmental treatment activities, the primary function of the splint is to help the therapist maintain the child's hand in the weight-bearing posture while facilitating proximal shoulder stability and active elbow extension. As proximal stability improves, the upper extremity will become free to develop equilibrium responses and higher-level manual skills. The child is encouraged to move more spontaneously through developmental patterns previously hampered by the flexed extremity. A secondary goal of the splint is to improve wrist and hand functions by elongating wrist and finger flexors while normalizing tone.

Indications

1. Children who lack adequate weight bearing and protective responses in the upper extremity(s) due to abnormal muscle tone

2. Children with mild to moderate hypotonia or hypertonia secondary to congenital and posttraumatic hemiplegia, mild diplegia, and selected cases of quadriplegia

3. Children with full or nearly full joint range—the splint is not designed to reduce contractures

4. Children with abnormal movement in the extremity as a result of spasticity rather than primitive reflexology such as a strong ATNR

Materials and construction (Figure 253)

1. A pattern is made which includes a volar support above the wrist joint and a rounded portion supporting the fingers and thumb.

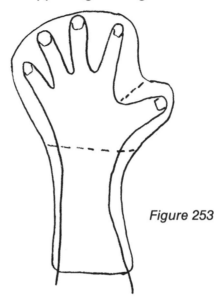

Figure 253

2. The splint is made of highly elastic LTT. The material is molded to the hand with an angle of 45 to 50 degrees of wrist extension.

3. The finger support is curved following the palmar arches with slight flexion of the PIP and DIP joints. This will help stimulate normal weight bearing in the hand and will provide relief for the tenodesis effect of tight finger flexors (Figure 254).

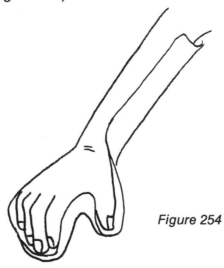

Figure 254

4. Strapping can be added, loose enough to allow for some movement within the splint as weight shifting is practiced.

Correct fit
1. Weight is borne on the heel of the hand with slight flexion of the IP joints of the fingers.

2. The thumb is positioned in abduction as tolerated.

3. The hand support extends to the end of the fingertips. Improper length of the hand support may cause irregular weight bearing.

Alternate fit
To accommodate more spontaneous weight shifting, the wrist support can be eliminated in cases of more mild spasticity. The splint should end distal to the distal crease of the wrist (Zahner 1985).

Precautions
A splint worn at times other than weight-bearing activities will inhibit the child's spontaneous upper-extremity extension and manipulative activities. Wearing of the splint should be gradually reduced to avoid dependence on it during weight bearing. Strapping should not inhibit the natural expansion of the hand during weight shifts.

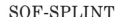

SOF-SPLINT

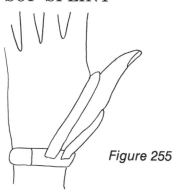

Figure 255

History and design rationale
The Sof-Splint was developed by Janet Reymann, out of a need to inhibit thumb retraction (marked flexion and adduction) in children with cortical brain damage (Reymann 1985). It was designed as a quick-to-fabricate, versatile, and inexpensive alternative to traditional LTT thumb abductor splints.

The splint is made from a form of neoprene material called Neo-Plush. It resembles a ⅛" thick piece of rubber-like material covered with nylon lining on one side and terry pile (velcro loop material) on the other side. The material has been used by medical and chiropractic practitioners as ankle, wrist, and knee supports. According to the designer, Neo-Plush is preferred over other strapping due to its stable yet elastic and dynamic properties. The flexibility of the material helps prevent pressure sores. Because of its dynamic properties, it encourages more active use of the hand during functional activities.

Unlike the one-piece thumb loop, adjustment of the thumb abduction strap is separate from the wrist strap. This allows for greater gradation in thumb position. For instance, the thumb strap can be placed on the radial side of the thumb and then gradually moved toward the dorsum of the wrist to grade the amount of thumb abduction and wrist extension. The strapping is designed to cross over the thenar eminence for prolonged deep pressure onto the muscle belly. Theoretically, this can have an inhibitory effect on thumb retraction.

Among other positive features of the Sof-Splint, it allows sensory exposure of the palm and maximizes the area available in the palm for grasp. It has a positive effect on the tactile and proprioceptive systems so the individual can remember how the thumb feels in the improved position. A carryover effect of increased thumb abduction has been reported lasting 20 minutes or longer after splint removal. Long-term effects reported include the acquisition of active wrist extension and thumb abduction.

Indications
1. Individuals with marked thumb adduction, secondary to hypertonus and resulting from cortical brain damage

2. Most effective with children but can be worn by the adolescent or adult with mild spasticity

3. May be more cosmetically acceptable than some other LTT splints

4. Some individuals with a mixture of athetosis and spasticity

5. Not recommended for patients with severe spasticity, contractures, or distal instability

6. Guarded use with infants or young children with small hands, due to the difficulty of fitting it correctly

7. Can be used in treatment when your direct facilitation on your patient's hand interferes with function. It is also helpful when the therapist's hands are needed elsewhere on the patient's body.

Materials
1. Two straps of Neo-Plush

2. Three pieces of velcro hook

Construction (Figure 256)
1. Cut the first strap to form a wrist band. The length of this piece is dependent upon the diameter of the wrist. The width is dependent upon the length of the forearm and the degree of wrist flexion exhibited by the patient. The terry pile (velcro loop) surface faces out.

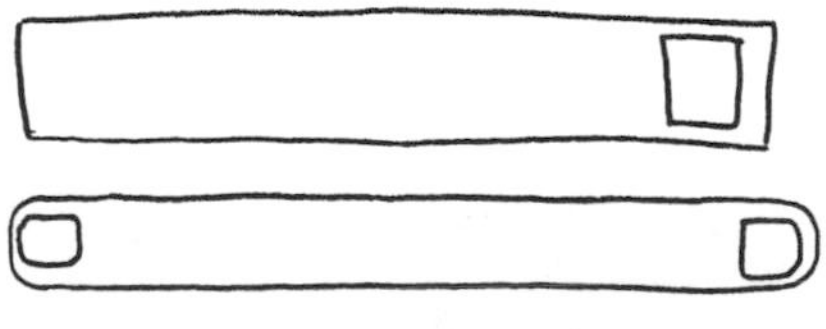

Figure 256

2. A small piece of velcro hook is sewn to one end of the strap on the nylon lining side, allowing easy fastening of the wrist strap to itself.

3. Cut a second strap to form the thumb band. The length and width will depend on the size of the hand. A piece of velcro hook sewn to each end allows this strap to attach to the wrist band. It should be pulled dorsal to volar to dorsal, across the thenar eminence and through the web space. The two ends of the strap attach next to one another on the dorsum of the wrist. This strap is pulled with sufficient tension to position the thumb in partial abduction and opposition. It can be graded according to need and tolerance.

Precautions

1. Incorrect donning above the MP joint will cause hyperextension at the IP joint of the thumb. For this reason, small children and infants may be difficult to fit.

2. Watch that the wrist is not pulled into excessive extension, especially when wearing at night.

3. The material can overstretch slightly after repeated use and will require frequent adjustment or replacement of the thumb strap. The strapping will lose its ability to adhere to velcro closure after repeated use, requiring replacement of the wrist strap. Worn daily, the life of the splint is three to six months.

Correct fit

The thumb strap fits comfortably in the web space, stretching across the thenar eminence and fastening both ends on the dorsum of the wrist band. Sufficient tension is used to facilitate thumb abduction and, if so indicated, wrist extension. The thumb band is maintained proximal to the head of the first MP joint, drawing the thumb into partial abduction and opposition.

Alternate fit

To facilitate a pincher grasp, pull the thumb strap across the PIP joints of the middle, ring, and little fingers so that these fingers are held flexed into the palm. Both ends of the strap will attach to the dorsal aspect of the wrist band as described previously in Figure 255. The strapping is returned to its original attachment when pinch activities are completed.

You may want to position the strapping between the fingers. This may facilitate an abduction and extension pattern. Wrist extension also can be facilitated by attaching the strap on the dorsum of the wrist band and drawing it through the first web space and across the palm.

Dynamic Splints

Dynamic orthoses employ moving parts such as rubber bands, tension wires, springs, or elastic-like materials. The splint is designed to correct or compensate for muscle imbalance, to increase range of motion and to improve joint alignment in the wrist and hand.

ORTHOKINETIC WRIST SPLINT

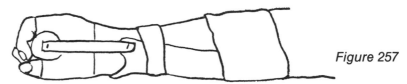

Figure 257

History and design rationale
The orthokinetic splint was developed by A. Joy Huss and adapted by Judith Hunt Kiel, incorporating the neurophysiological principals of Rood. Several mechanisms are employed to decrease flexor hypertonicity:

1. A hard cone placed in the hand presses on the insertion of wrist and hand flexors, concurrently inhibiting the extrinsic flexor muscles and reciprocally facilitating the extensor muscle groups.

2. The forearm shell acts as a further inhibiting force by providing maintained pressure onto the volar arm surface.

3. Three elastic straps (orthokinetic cuffs), securing the forearm shell in place, offer tactile stimulation to the extensor surface of the forearm, thus facilitating extensor activity.

No data on the effectiveness of this splint have been published or are known to the author.

Indications
Farber recommends the splint for patients with flexor hypertonicity who have at least minimal voluntary extension in the upper extremities (Farber and Huss 1974).

Materials and construction
The forearm shell, made of low-temperature thermoplastics (LTT), extends two-thirds the length of the forearm, volar aspect. The shell starts approximately 3 cm from the wrist crease. The hand piece, also fabricated of plastic, is shaped into a cone. The smaller end of the cone is directed radially with a thumb groove recommended to alleviate pressure in the web space. Two side supports attach the forearm piece to the cone. The side supports are loosely riveted in place, allowing the wrist to move freely.

Correct fit
The wrist hinge of the splint should be in alignment with the wrist joint of the arm.

Precautions
The splint may be contraindicated in cases of the fisted hand, thumb-in-palm deformities, and severe ulnar or radial deviation. Lining the splint with soft foam may facilitate flexors and, in addition, may cause skin breakdown secondary to heat and moisture retention by the foam.

MACKINNON SPLINT

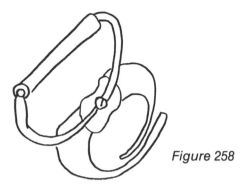

Figure 258

History and design rationale
This dynamic splint was designed by MacKinnon in 1973 to improve hand function in children with spastic cerebral palsy (MacKinnon, Sanderson, and Buchanan 1975). The splint was modified by Exner and Bonder (1983) who enlarged the LTT piece for the dorsum of the forearm and added an additional strap for increased stability. Without this modification, the LTT piece tended to slide onto the dorsum of the hand. A wooden dowel placed in the palm of the hand was designed to provide pressure to the MC heads and stretch to the intrinsics. This inhibited the finger flexors and reduced spasticity. Relatively nonrestrictive, the splint allows for sensory input into the palm.

MacKinnon and colleagues reported increased awareness and use of the involved hand in children, one to five years of age, with spastic-type hemiplegia. They noted decreased fisting of the hand with more frequent thumb abduction as a result of wearing the splint. Exner and Bonder compared the MacKinnon splint with a short opponens splint and orthokinetic cuff. They reported that the MacKinnon splint was most often associated with improvement in grasp and bilateral hand use.

Indications
1. Strong associated movements and reactions in the hand that interfere with function
2. Spasticity that is present all the time
3. Spasticity that is present with voluntary movement
4. Hand disregard
5. Flexor tone and poor wrist alignment

Materials and construction (Figure 259)
1. Use wooden or LTT doweling, ¼" to ½" in diameter and the width of the child's hand. It is sufficient in size to contact the MC heads without interfering with hand function. A firm pad can be added to the radial end of the dowel to increase thumb abduction.

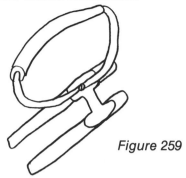

Figure 259

2. Obtain latex tubing, such as catheter or aquarium tubing, ⅛" to ¼" in diameter. Attach the tubing to either end of the dowel with small wood screws, tacks, or nails that have flat heads. When using LTT instead of a wooden dowel, form the MC piece around the tubing, creating one continuous piece.

3. A small kidney-shaped or larger I-shaped piece of LTT fits on the dorsum of the forearm above the wrist crease. The tubing and velcro wrist straps are anchored to this forearm piece via a sleeve screw or rivet. The tubing can be shortened on the radial side to help control ulnar drift. Feel free to experiment with different wrist band designs.

Correct fit
1. The wrist should not be forced into a functional position. Dorsiflexion of 15 degrees is the maximum range desired for functional use of the hand.

2. The palmar bar is maintained at the MC heads and is small enough to avoid impeding movement at the distal palmar crease.

Precautions
1. Use of a wood dowel is contraindicated with young children who may mouth and chew the splint.

2. The wood dowel tends to "flatten" the palm. LTT curved to support the arch of the hand may be preferred.

3. It is difficult to keep the dowel from slipping away from the MC heads and into the palm. This may reduce the area of the palm available for holding objects, particularly when the finger flexors are tight.

4. The upper extremity is carefully monitored for changes in tone. As the splint reduces spasticity, the hand can develop hypotonicity. The shoulder may become unstable as well.

5. Watch for pressure to the ulnar styloid caused by the wrist band.

DYNAMIC WRIST AND ARCH SUPPORT
WITH THUMB OPPONENS OR "J SPLINT"

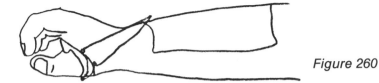

Figure 260

History and design rationale

I designed this splint as part of a research study that explored the efficacy of splinting children with spasticity secondary to cerebral palsy. The splint borrows the basic idea behind the MacKinnon splint. The "J splint" is named for the shape of the thumb support pattern. It utilizes a dynamic force at the wrist to facilitate wrist alignment and extension while putting pressure into the palm and web space to relax the hand and increase its availability for function.

Unlike the MacKinnon splint, the palmar bar rests below the head of the MP joints and is curved rather than flat, to support the transverse arch. The bar extends on the radial side, encircling the thumb in a J-shaped configuration which supports the first MP joint and rotates the thumb into abduction and opposition.

Several considerations contributed to the design. The placement of a foam-lined forearm trough on the dorsum of the arm stimulates the extensor musculature beneath. The use of the dynamic traction applied to the wrist encourages more active alignment of the wrist and passively stretches the wrist flexors. When positioned correctly, the J-shaped configuration has a unique ability to press into the palm to support the longitudinal arch as it provides pressure on the lateral border of the thenar eminence, inhibiting thumb adductors.

The splint is meant to be worn for 10 to 15 minutes during prehension, drawing, or free play, following a period of exercise. Functional activities are continued after the splint is removed. Through positioning, verbal cues, and other feedback, the child is encouraged to carry over the sensory effect of the orthosis. Generally speaking, when the splint works, a change in resting position and function will be observed almost immediately with the splint on. It is most helpful for aligning the wrist in children who have voluntary wrist extension but lack radial deviation during activity. In at least one case, a child who was developing radial deviation began playing with a greater combination of wrist and forearm movements with the splint on than was previously seen.

One major drawback of the splint is the tendency for distal excursion by the forearm trough. For this reason, the splint may need to be repositioned several times within a treatment session. Another problem with the splint design is the angle of pull by the traction device. The force potential is not optimized at a 90-degree angle. Like any other orthotic device, the "J splint" is meant to be used as an adjunct to therapy and serves as a key point of control during functional activities.

Indications
1. For children with mild to moderate spasticity who have voluntary wrist extension, approximately 20 degrees or more, but lack sufficient stability to maintain radial deviation during grasp and release

2. May work best in cases of hemiplegia. In cases of bilateral involvement, I recommend one splint be worn at a time.

Materials
1. Use an LTT of your choice. I prefer using materials with controlled stretch for the spastic hand.

2. ⅛" closed-cell soft foam lining

3. Five small dress hooks

4. Assorted rubber bands

5. 2" wide velcro loop strapping

6. Two pieces of self-adhesive velcro hook, each approximately 2" long

Construction
1. Construct the dorsal-based forearm trough. Measure the length from the ulnar styloid to two-thirds the length of the forearm. The width reaches from the midline of the lateral border to the midline of the medial border. Flare the material at the ulnar styloid as well as the proximal and distal ends. Round and smooth all edges.

2. Line the forearm trough with self-adhesive foam and add velcro closures.

3. Fasten a dress hook to the distal end of the trough at the midline. The opening of the hook is directed toward the elbow.

4. Develop the pattern for the J-shaped arch and thumb support (Figure 261). You may wish to use pieces of masking tape applied directly to the skin or pieces of paper taped together for the patient with sensitive skin.

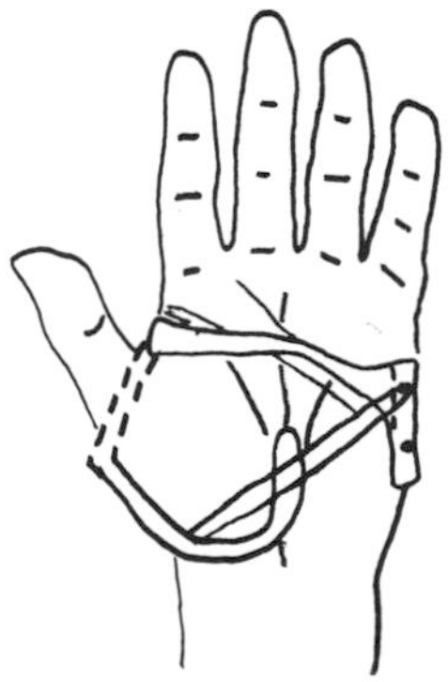

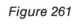

Figure 261

a. Fit the ulnar border support using a 1″ to 1½″ square of paper on the palm below the distal (palmar) transverse crease, fastening it around to the dorsum of the hand.

b. Add a thin strip of paper to the ulnar border support and place it in the palm, following the natural curve between the proximal and distal transverse creases. This palmar bar will become the transverse arch support in the splint.

c. The next piece added fits within the web space. The size may vary depending on the amount of thumb adduction displayed. It is critical to fit the pattern comfortably below the proximal transverse arch. For the patient who needs more support, position it ½″ above this crease to have a C-bar effect.

d. To the web spacer described above, add the hook of the J so that it encircles the thumb for support to the first MP joint.

e. Bring this piece down and around the thenar eminence as you passively rotate the thumb into the desired position of abduction and opposition.

f. Add a final piece of paper between the thenar crease and the middle palmar crease. This part of the splint will serve as the longitudinal arch support. The material ends at a point parallel with the first MP joint.

5. It is advisable to press the tape firmly together before removing the patterns from the patient's hand. Immediately transfer the pattern to a solid piece of paper and check it for fit, making any corrections to the pattern before using the splint material.

6. Transfer the pattern onto the splint material. Heat and cut the pattern. Reheat to ensure proper contouring during fabrication.

7. Fit the thumb and arch support on the hand in the same order as the pattern was made. The hook of the J is the most difficult part of the splint to fit and will take several attempts to fit correctly (Figure 262). It helps to rotate the thumb into abduction and opposition as you place the material around the thumb and press it between the thenar and middle palmar creases. Allow the material to harden.

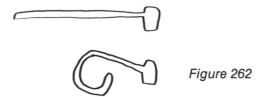

Figure 262

8. Round and smooth all edges.

9. Add two dress hooks to the ulnar border so they are placed parallel with the fifth metacarpal. These can be heated and secured into place using additional splinting material. The opening of the hook should face the volar aspect of the hand (hook #1 = distal, hook #2 = proximal).

10. Fasten the last two dress hooks to the radial border of the thumb and arch support so that one hook (hook #3 = distal) is parallel with the head of the first metacarpal and the other hook (hook #4 = proximal) is placed close to its base. These hooks open toward the volar aspect of the hand.

11. Be sure the splint material is completely cooled and hardened before proceeding. Approaching the splint from the palm, attach a rubber band from hook #4 to hook #1. This placement may seem awkward since the hooks will be opening the "wrong way." This placement of this rubber band is necessary to help press the splint into the longitudinal arch.

12. Attach a rubber band from hooks #1 and #2 to the hook on the forearm trough and another rubber band from hooks #3 and #4 to the forearm trough. The length of the rubber bands will be determined by the amount of wrist extension desired. No further strapping should be needed.

Correct fit

1. The key to fitting this splint is to build good arch supports, both transverse and longitudinal, utilizing the creases of the palm as natural guidelines for placement of the splint material.

2. The base of the first MP joint should be supported in a stable position.

3. Reinforcing the developmental sequence, the thumb can be supported in an abducted and extended position to encourage lateral prehension. The thumb is gradually rotated into abduction and opposition for the development of finer prehension.

4. It is important to place the hook of the J between the thenar crease and the middle palmar crease so that it presses into the longitudinal arch, not into the thenar eminence.

5. Allow a space, approximately ½", between the transverse arch and longitudinal arch supports. This will help accommodate movement in the palm.

6. Consider utilizing an ulnar gutter in place of the dorsal-based forearm trough. This may help prevent migration of the forearm piece in some cases.

Precautions

1. Watch for pressure areas, particularly at the web space and ulnar styloid.

2. A child with tight finger flexors may need wrist positioning closer to neutral. Adjust the rubber band tension accordingly.

3. It may be difficult to keep the forearm trough in place. Adjust as needed; however, watch that the straps are not excessively tight.

4. Watch for hyperextension at the IP joints. You can correct this problem by having the patient wear PIP flexion splints in conjunction with the J splint.

5. Limit the wearing time to 10 to 15 minutes following exercise. Follow splint removal with a feedback period in which new wrist and palmar activity are reinforced. Offer the patient unfamiliar objects and activities to encourage new patterns of movement.

References to Appendix A

Blashy, M., and R. Fuchs. 1959. Orthokinetics: A new receptor facilitation method. *American Journal of Occupational Therapy* 13:226.

Bloch, R., and M. Evans. 1977. An inflatable splint for the spastic hand. *Archives of Physical Medicine and Rehabilitation* 58:179-180.

Bobath, B. 1971. *Adult hemiplegia: Evaluation and treatment.* London: William Heinemann Medical Books, Ltd.

Bobath, B., and K. Bobath. 1964. The facilitation of normal postural reactions and movements in the treatment of cerebral palsy. *Physiotherapy* 8:3-19.

_____ . 1975. *Motor development in the different types of cerebral palsy.* London: William Heineman Medical Books, Ltd.

Brennan, J. 1959. Response to stretch of hypertonic muscle groups in hemiplegia. *British Medical Journal* 1:1504-1507.

Brunnstrom, S. 1956. Associated reactions of the upper extremity in adult patients with hemiplegia: An approach to training. *Physical Therapy Review* 36:225-236.

Cannon, N. 1985. *Manual of hand splinting.* New York: Churchill Livingstone.

Charait, S. 1968. A comparison of volar and dorsal splinting of the hemiplegic hand. *American Journal of Occupational Therapy* 22:319-321.

Doubilet, L., and L. Polkow. 1977. Theory and design of a finger abduction splint for the spastic hand. *American Journal of Occupational Therapy* 31:320-322.

Erhardt, R. 1982. *Developmental hand dysfunction: Theory, assessment, treatment.* Laurel, MD: Ramsco Publishing Co.

Exner, C., and B. Bonder. 1983. Comparative effects of three hand splints on the bilateral hand use, grasp, and arm-hand posture in hemiplegic children: A pilot study. *The Occupational Therapy Journal of Research* 3:75-92.

Farber, S., and A. Huss. 1974. *Sensorimotor evaluation and treatment procedure for allied health.* Indiana: Purdue University Press.

Fess, E., K. Gettle, and J. Strickland. 1981. *Hand splinting: Principles and methods.* St. Louis, MO: C.V. Mosby.

Gesell, A., and A. Amatruda. 1949. *Developmental diagnosis.* New York: Harper and Row.

Greenberg, S., and R. Braun. 1977. Therapeutic uses of the air bag splint for the injured hand. *American Journal of Occupational Therapy* 31:318-319.

Grossman, M., S. Sahrmann, and S. Rose. 1982. Review of length-associated changes in muscle: Experimental evidence and clinical implications. *Physical Therapy* 62:12.

Hill, S. 1985. Splinting program for children with upper extremity spasticity secondary to cerebral palsy. Unpublished paper.

Hunter, J., L. Schneider, E. Mackin, and J. Bell, eds. 1983. *Rehabilitation of the hand,* 2nd ed. St. Louis, MO: C.V. Mosby.

Jamison, S., and N. Dayhoff. 1980. A hard hand-positioning device to decrease wrist and finger hypertonicity: A sensorimotor approach for the patient with nonprogressive brain damage. *Nursing Research* 29:5.

Johnstone, M. 1975. Inflatable splint for the hemiplegic arm. *Physiotherapy* 61:377.

————— . 1978. *Restoration of motor function in the stroke patient.* Edinburgh: Churchill Livingstone.

Kaplan, N. 1962. Effects of splinting on reflex inhibition and sensorimotor stimulation in treatment of spasticity. *Archives of Physical Medicine and Rehabilitation* 43:565-569.

Lindholm, L. 1985. Weight-bearing splint: A method for managing upper extremity spasticity. *Physical Therapy Forum* 5:3.

MacKinnon, J., E. Sanderson, and J. Buchanan. 1975. The MacKinnon Splint—a functional hand splint. *Canadian Journal of Occupational Therapy* 42:157-158.

Malick, M. 1980. *Manual on static hand splinting,* Vol. 1, 4th ed. Pittsburgh: Harmarville Rehabilitation Center.

McPherson, J. 1981. Objective evaluation of a splint designed to reduce hypertonicty. *American Journal of Occupational Therapy* 53:189-194.

McPherson, J., D. Kreimeyer, M. Aaderks, and T. Gallagher. 1980. A comparison of dorsal and volar resting hand splints in the reduction of hypertonus. *American Journal of Occuptional Therapy* 36:664-670.

Mills, V. 1984. Electromyographic results of inhibitory splinting. *Physical Therapy* 64:190-193.

Neuhaus, B., E. Ascher, B. Coullon, M. Donohue, A. Einbond, J. Glover, S. Goldberg, and V. Takai. 1981. A survey of rationales for and against hand splinting in hemiplegia. *American Journal of Occupational Therapy* 35:83-95.

Reymann, J. 1985. The sof-splint. *Developmental Disabilities Newsletter of the American Occupational Therapy Association* 8:2.

Rood, M. 1954. Neurophysiological reactions as a basis for physical therapy. *Physical Therapy Review* 34:444-449.

Snook, J. 1981. Spasticity reduction splint. *American Journal of Occupational Therapy* 33:648-651.

Trombly, C. 1983. *Occupational therapy for physical dysfunction.* 2nd ed. Baltimore, MD: Williams and Wilkins.

Zahner, K. March 12, 1985. Personal communication.

Zizlis, J. 1964. Splinting of the hand in a spastic hemiplegic patient. *Archives of Physical Medicine and Rehabilitation* 1:41-43.

Acknowledgments—Appendix A

I would like to thank the following people for helping make this written material possible:

Jan Dobbs, Pat Harkansee, and Pam Miller
of Smith and Nephew Rolyan Incorporated

Susanne Higgins, Charlotte Exner, Janet Reynman, and Jan Utley
for reviewing the content

Joyce Dawnie, Kathy Serikaku, Kris Razma, Kathleen Zahner
for suggestions regarding splinting

Luz Giren,
for typing and editing

Coleen O'Connell,
for her friendship and support throughout this project

About the Author of Appendix A

Susan Hill is a graduate of the University of Illinois and holds a B.S. degree in occupational therapy. She has specialized in pediatrics for the past twelve years. Susan is currently employed as a senior therapist at Gilchrist Marchman Rehabilitation Center and is a private consultant in the Chicago area. In 1985 Susan developed and implemented "A splint program for children with upper extremity spasticity secondary to cerebral palsy," funded by the National Easter Seal Research Foundation.

Casting to Improve Upper Extremity Function

Audrey Yasukawa, MOT, OTR/L
Judy Hill, BSOT, OTR/L

Spasticity and imbalances of muscle function around a joint, resulting in synergistic or patterned motion, are common in the upper extremities—indeed the entire bodies—of neurologically impaired patients. The disorders of muscle tonus limit the repertoire of movements available and subsequently interfere with functional use of the extremities. Secondary problems can also develop as a result of persistent spasticity or rigidity. These include circulatory changes when vessels are constricted by tight muscles or joint structures, muscle and soft tissue contracture, and orthopedic problems.

Indications for Casting

Occupational therapy management of the neurologically impaired upper extremity must address both the primary and secondary problems observed in motor disorders associated with spasticity. Treatment principles which address as many of the component problems as possible should be incorporated into management techniques.

Treatment principles in spasticity management include (1) slow, gentle, nonabrupt movement to avoid setting off stretch reflexes; (2) the maintenance of muscle length through relaxation; (3) the incorporation of positions which seem to have a relaxing effect on other joints of the extremity; and (4) the incorporation of the more relaxed muscle state and joint position into functional movement. Where problems such as muscle and soft tissue contracture have occurred secondary to abnormal tone, treatment techniques may include gentle, prolonged stretch, allowing tissues to expand through cell division as opposed to being stretched during intermittent periods of time. Stretching tissues, by applying too great a mechanical pressure too quickly, can actually cause tearing of tissues and result in scarring and further loss of elasticity. Circulatory problems and edema that are caused by constriction require mobilization of fluids, elevation, and reversing factors contributing to the constriction. Once fixed orthopedic problems develop secondary to the pull exerted by spastic muscles, surgical realignment may be necessary. If intervention can be made before the deformity becomes fixed, realignment may be improved by reducing the pull of spastic or contracted muscles and supporting the joint position.

Rationale

Inhibitory, serial casts provide prolonged, gentle stretch to spastic or contracted muscles. They can also support the upper extremity joints with improved joint alignment and position. Casts are positioned statically in a submaximal range to avoid elicitation of the stretch reflex. Submaximal range is defined as 5 to 10 degrees less than the range available with maximal stretch. The cast protects the limb from external stimuli which could set off reflex activity.

Inhibitory casts are those used to reduce the effects of abnormal tone by placing muscles in a position that has a relaxing effect on them. Casting one portion of the arm may also have a relaxing effect on other muscles in that extremity. For example, casting a thumb in extension may relax finger flexors. Casting the forearm in supination may have an inhibitory effect on spasticity in the elbow, wrist, or hand.

Serial casting procedures are based on the biomechanics of muscle length. For example, the arm may be bound by elbow flexion and forearm supination as a result of a biceps contracture. A series of casts placing the limb in successively greater ranges of elbow extension and forearm pronation can be used to reverse the biceps contracture. While the spastic or contracted muscles are maintained in a gradually more lengthened range, their antagonists are maintained in a shortened range, facilitating their activity when the cast is removed.

General Protocol

Casts are applied in a series, with each cast being left in place for three to seven days, depending on the severity of tone and type of cast. When one cast in the series is removed, another is applied immediately following cleansing of the extremity, examination of the skin for pressure areas, and assessment of range of motion and muscle tone. The intervention series is generally limited to five to seven casts in order to prevent excessive stiffness and promote the incorporation of gains made with casting into functional movement. The last cast may be bivalved, or cut into two halves, with the seams or edges finished. The bivalve cast is used intermittently to maintain the gains made in range of motion and improved muscle tone. Active facilitation techniques are utilized to incorporate these gains into functional movement.

The limb's response to the casting series is not always predictable. There may be improvement but, perhaps, not as much as you had hoped for. The casting program is still discontinued after the seventh cast and is replaced by aggressive facilitation for upper extremity function. However, another cast series may be utilized at a later date to further influence range of motion and tone.

Improvement should be observed by the time the second cast is removed. When range of motion has not increased by more than 5 degrees, or reduction in tone and/or improvement in volitional movement are not seen, the casting program is interrupted. The second cast is bivalved and used to maintain range of motion while other treatment methods are used to maintain mobility. If changes in spontaneous motion are noted at a later date, the casting program may be reinstated.

In cases of rigidity, where the limb is maintained in a fixed position and attempts at passive movement in either direction meet with significant resistance, casting may be contraindicated. Treatment for rigidity attempts to widen the arc of available range, increasing mobility. Static positioning for five to seven days could actually contribute to an increase in stiffness. Alternating bivalved casts, with one positioned in submaximal flexion and the other in submaximal extension, may be used in these cases to reduce the tone and gradually increase the joint movement at the end of both ranges.

Principles of Casting

Casts are fabricated to enclose, either fully or partially, joints acted on by spastic muscles along with the areas proximal and distal to those joints. As much surface area as possible is enclosed in each cast to achieve maximum pressure distribution and to position the extremity and support the joint as fully as possible. A cast that is too short decreases the available leverage and results in pressure points at the proximal and distal ends of the cast. Casts are fabricated from stockinette and cotton cast padding covered with plaster gauze. When a cast is intended to be used as a bivalved splint for maintenance, fiberglass casting materials are often used instead of plaster for increased durability. Cast application requires two therapists, one to position the limb while the cast is applied and the other to apply the cast.

Assessment

Physician's orders are required prior to initiating a casting program. The physician may use x-rays to rule out orthopedic causes for the immobility or those conditions which may contraindicate the use of casting such as heterotopic ossification, with its presenting symptoms of inflammation and stiffness. Patients with open wounds and severe edema are not casted.

Once the medical referral is received, the entire extremity is evaluated, including joints proximal and distal to those being casted. Casting can have an effect, either positive or negative, on joints adjacent to the site of casting. This is particularly true when the cast is impacting on muscles that cross over more than one joint. The cast has the potential to affect a second joint crossed by a muscle, at the same time that it affects the casted joint.

For example, when casting a contracted elbow toward extension, the gleno-humeral joint could exhibit reduced external rotation range as the biceps muscle is slowly stretched at the elbow.

Pre- and postcast series evaluation will include goniometric evaluation of single joint range of motion with consideration for total muscle length. For example, limitations of long finger flexor length are isolated from wrist limitation by measuring wrist extension with fingers both flexed and extended. Spasticity is evaluated using goniometric measurement of the point at which the stretch reflex is elicited and by timing the patient's ability to perform rapid alternating motions. Upper extremity sensation is documented and can be an indicator of projected functional outcomes.

The patient's arm placement at rest and during general movement is observed. Since the ultimate goal of casting is to improve upper extremity control, a functional assessment is also important. This would include active placing and holding of the arm in space, use of the elbow to functionally shorten and lengthen the extremity, use of forearm and wrist to alter the hand position in space, and the ability of the hand to grasp and release objects. Between each cast in a series, range of motion of the joint casted and spasticity are reassessed. Each cast is marked with the date of application and projected removal date.

Cast Monitoring

The newly casted extremity is monitored hourly for several hours, by comparing the casted to the uncasted extremity. The temperature and pulse of the casted extremity is compared to the uncasted extremity. Skin coloration is compared for dusky veins and nail beds. A grayish coloration may indicate circulatory problems. The extremity is examined for significant edema. Mild edema may occur two to three hours post cast application, especially in the fingers if they have been used by the holder to position the limb during cast application.

Pressure areas may be a problem at the distal and proximal borders of the cast. One finger should insert easily and two fingers snugly into the distal and proximal ends of the cast. A cast that is too tight can constrict nerves and vessels. A cast that is too loose can allow slippage, causing skin abrasion, and will not adequately support the joint.

The patient may report pain or other changes in sensation. Slight discomfort or a "pulling" sensation is often present and expected. Problems in any of the above signs may indicate the need for immediate removal of the cast. When casting outpatients, the patient or a family member must be taught to monitor the cast and to have the cast removed if any problems occur.

Factors that Influence Outcome

In the neurologically impaired patient, there are a number of factors which seem to influence the results of casting. The more motor control the patient has prior to casting, the greater the therapeutic gains postcasting. The greater the degree of patterned versus isolated motion, the more difficult it will be to maintain newly gained range. When spastic proximal motor function persists, distal motor disorders tend to recur following casting even when significant gains have been made in motor function during the casting program.

The longer a spastic pattern or contracture has existed, the more difficult it seems to be to correct. For example, a wrist flexion contracture which has persisted for many years will have resulted in loss of elasticity of the flexor muscles, secondary soft tissue contractures, overstretch of extensor musculature, and possible malalignment of the carpal bones. These factors will impact on the outcome of the casting intervention. The longer the patient has been relying on abnormal motor patterns and compensatory movements to function, the more difficult those patterns are to influence.

Sensation and unilateral neglect will negatively impact on the functional results of casting, just as they influence functional use of an extremity. Cognitive status and the patient's ability to participate in an active therapy program with the cast in place will also influence the results of casting and the carryover into function.

The goals of a casting program can vary from improving the resting position of the extremity for cosmesis and hygiene to making functional movement possible. Goals are set based on the pre-cast assessment and factors described above which influence the results of casting.

Types of Casts and Criteria for Use

Common clinical presentations of upper extremity dysfunction in neurologically impaired patients include internal rotation with abduction or adduction of the humerus, forearm posturing in an extreme rotational range, and the flexion-bound elbow, wrist, and hand. From the initial assessment of the client, the therapist will be responsible for choosing the type of cast to best enhance function with each type of clinical presentation. The various types of casts will be described with considerations for use and contraindications. There are no strict rules as to which cast to use, but utilizing general guidelines and principles will be helpful in the decision-making process. The therapist must rely on clinical judgment, experience, and problem-solving skills. Once the casting series is terminated, ongoing monitoring and aggressive treatment of the extremity are essential to assist the patient in maintaining and functionally using the new alignment and range.

DROP-OUT CAST: HUMERUS ENCLOSED

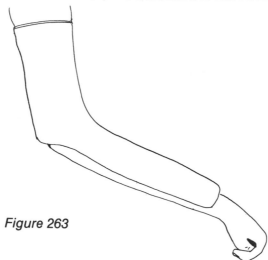

Figure 263

Indications

The drop-out cast with the humeral portion enclosed has been most effective for an individual with severe elbow flexion contracture.

Effects

1. It can increase elbow range quickly and the additional range can be seen as it occurs, since the partially enclosed portion of the limb drops away from the cast. As the forearm drops out of the cast, an increase of about 10 to 15 degrees of elbow extension will indicate the need for a new cast.

2. The forearm shell prevents flexion of the arm and maintains range.

3. When the patient is sitting in an upright position, the pull of gravity will assist with elbow extension.

4. Since the open portion of the forearm shell allows the elbow to drop out, the patient and/or therapist can facilitate passive and/or active movement.

5. Previous skin breakdown in the forearm may require the arm to be left exposed.

Contraindications

1. Heterotopic ossification of the joint is usually managed by active and/ or passive range of motion rather than casting.

2. The drop-out cast will not provide sustained positioning to control the type of extremity where fluctuations in muscle tone quickly change from very low to very high.

3. Attempts to fabricate the drop-out cast for an elbow with a minimal elbow extension contracture have not been successful due to slippage. The rigid circular elbow cast is recommended for minimal range of motion limitations.

DROP-OUT CAST: FOREARM ENCLOSED

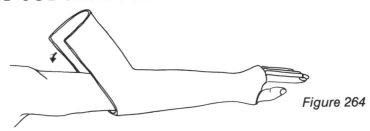

Figure 264

Indications
The forearm-enclosed drop-out cast can incorporate the wrist and forearm while increasing range at the elbow. This cast can be applied on a patient with skin breakdown in the humeral region.

Effects
1. The humeral shell prevents flexion of the arm and maintains range.

2. By including the forearm and wrist, the position may assist with decreasing the tone at the elbow joint. The cast will position the forearm and wrist statically, providing a slow stretch at the elbow. The flexors of the elbow gradually elongate without overstretching the joints.

3. By incorporating the wrist, contractures in forearm rotation can be gently controlled.

Contraindications
1. Heterotopic ossification

2. Fluctuating tone

3. This cast is awkward for the patient to wear. Patients may complain of difficulty with donning and doffing clothes and wearing shirts comfortably.

REVERSE DROP-OUT CAST

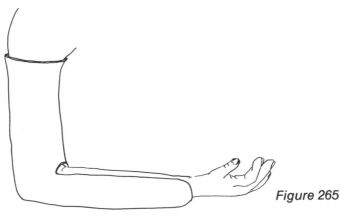

Figure 265

Indications

The reverse drop-out cast is used when spasticity has created an extension contracture with decreased range in elbow flexion.

Effects

1. It gradually increases range into elbow flexion.

2. It places the weak biceps at a mechanical advantage to work.

Contraindications

1. Heterotopic ossification

2. Fluctuating tone

RIGID CIRCULAR ELBOW CAST

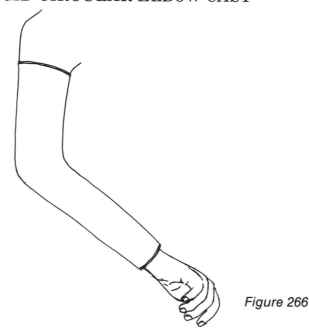

Figure 266

Indications

The rigid circular elbow cast can be applied on a patient to gradually increase elbow range. It may be used with fluctuating tone, since the cast can provide equalized pressure throughout the arm. This stabilizing effect will neutralize the impact of the abnormal muscle tone, allowing for a gradual increase in elbow range.

Effects

1. It is one of the preferred approaches to the severely spastic arm. Again the equalized pressure has a tendency to reduce the impact of the tone on the extremity.

2. It can be used on an elbow with a minimal to moderate contracture because, when properly fitted, it will not slide.

Contraindications

1. Heterotopic ossification

2. The cast is left on for five to seven days for the inhibitory effect to work; therefore, it is difficult to check for skin tolerance and possible breakdown.

3. Rigid muscle tone

LONG ARM CAST

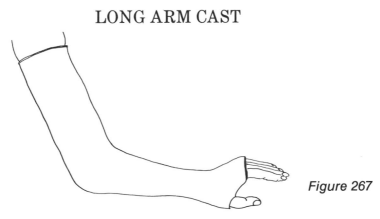

Figure 267

Indications

The long arm cast includes the elbow, forearm, and wrist. It is used to simultaneously manage problems at those joints. It is the only cast effective in controlling spastic pronator or supinator muscles.

Effects

1. By incorporating the wrist, supination and pronation contractures can be gently controlled.

2. The position of the forearm and wrist may assist with reducing overall tone and subsequently increasing range of motion throughout the upper extremity.

3. The long arm cast may reduce the dominance of the spasticity and rebalance the antagonistic motor group. This may then be a reasonable approach for patients who exhibit upper extremity motor function as a mass synergy pattern that involves simultaneous motion at each joint rather than a selective muscular control. Muscle re-education is important in facilitating isolated control, since muscle weakness is a common problem, especially in the extensor groups.

Contraindications

1. It is sometimes difficult to position the patient with severe flexor spasticity. The arm may not tolerate the force of the cast on multiple joints. Overstretching may cause skin breakdown or microtears in soft tissue.

2. Rigid muscle tone

3. Skin problems that may require that the arm be left exposed

WRIST CAST

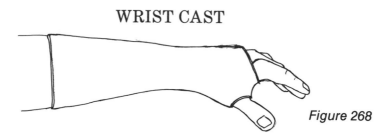

Figure 268

Indications

The rigid circular cast is indicated for the wrist that exhibits spasticity, contractures, and general weakness. The problems may be seen in isolation or in combination with involvement of other joints. This cast makes facilitation of functional movement possible by increasing range of wrist motion, reducing abnormal tone, and differentiating or isolating wrist from hand motion.

Effects

1. The cast can improve the position of the hand for skin care and hygiene.

2. It can improve the position and alignment of the severely involved hand. Eventually the hand can be properly fitted and maintained by a lightweight, low-temperature plastic splint.

3. The cast series can release movements previously hidden and dominated by marked spasticity. For example, by reducing wrist flexor tone, an improved balance between wrist flexion and extension is possible. The patient with limited active extension as a result of insufficient power may require a wrist orthosis after the casting program. The splint will assist with supporting the wrist, maintaining proper joint alignment and muscle length.

4. The cast can stabilize the wrist joint, creating the possibility of improvement in grasp, pinch, release, and manipulation. This cast is beneficial for patients who have difficulty coordinating wrist and finger movements. For example, as the patient attempts to extend the wrist, the metacarpophalangeal (MCP) joints may hyperextend (Figure 269). Swan neck or boutonniere deformities eventually may develop. This pattern is often associated with wrist instability. Weakness of the wrist extensors may complicate the situation. This muscle imbalance may be accompanied by spasticity of the intrinsic muscles. This type of cast can stabilize the wrist and maintain good alignment. It can provide the proximal stability at the wrist needed for distal control of the fingers. With the wrist in a proper position, the muscle imbalance seen at the fingers may correct itself.

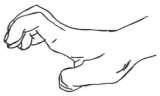

Figure 269

Contraindications

1. Edema in the hand

2. Subluxation of the carpal bones or other orthopedic deformities may require specialized therapeutic techniques or surgery.

METACARPOPHALANGEAL (MCP) WRIST CAST

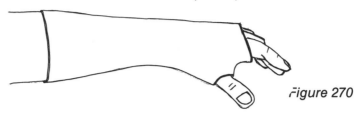

Figure 270

Indications

A wrist cast can be applied that incorporates the MCP joints. This type of cast is used when spasticity of the intrinsics causes flexion contractures of the MCP joints. This contracture can result in the intrinsic plus type hand, where the patient can only flex and extend the fingers with the MCP joints in flexion.

Effects

1. The cast can gradually extend the MCP joint into full extension.

2. The patient can have the opportunity to work actively on finger flexion and extension of the PIP and DIP joints while gradually elongating the intrinsic musculature.

Contraindications

1. Edema

2. Subluxation or other orthopedic deformities

WRIST CAST WITH THUMB ENCLOSED

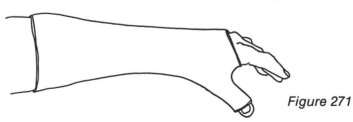

Figure 271

Indications

A wrist cast with the thumb enclosed can be utilized to manage the thumb-in-palm deformity caused by spasticity of the thumb flexor and adductor. This deformity prevents the thumb from participating in grasp and pinch. The spasticity and/or contracture of the thumb may cause secondary problems characterized by shortening of the web space, joint subluxation, an unstable MCP joint, or an overstretched extensor pollicis. A wrist cast with the thumb enclosed can be applied to enhance grasp or to improve overall range and tone of the hand.

Effects
1. Positioning of the thumb may have a relaxing effect on the spasticity in the fingers and wrist.

2. The position may elongate the thumb flexor and possibly improve the power of the thumb extensors.

Contraindications
1. Edema

2. Subluxation or other orthopedic deformities

FINGER SHELL

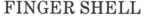

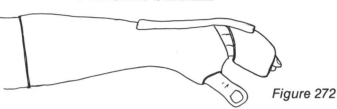

Figure 272

Indications
In severe flexion contractures of the wrist and fingers, function is greatly impaired. There is severe spasticity of the wrist flexors, as well as the finger flexors and the intrinsics. A finger shell can be attached to a wrist cast to provide a slow, gradual stretch of the fingers into extension.

Effects
1. Initially, the shell can be positioned with the MCP joint in flexion. As the fingers relax, the shell gradually can be pulled up into extension, providing the intrinsics with slow, careful, elongation of the muscle fibers.

2. It will improve position and muscle balance, enhancing the potential for distal function.

3. It will improve the position of the fingers for hygiene.

4. It will improve the position of the hand for eventual splinting.

5. The shell is removable which allows for gradual build-up of wearing tolerance and monitoring of the fingers for complications.

Contraindications
1. Circulation problems at the fingers

2. Severe spasticity in the fingers may cause potential microtearing of the soft tissues and small muscles of the hand due to improper fit and pull of the finger shell.

PLATFORM CAST

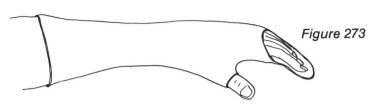

Figure 273

Indications
The platform cast is used with minimal spasticity. The patient generally exhibits isolated muscle control, but continues to be influenced by the mild flexor tone. The increased tone causes a muscle imbalance which interferes with efficient and precise small muscle blend patterns. When the patient attempts to extend the wrist and fingers, slight flexion of the long finger flexors and thumb flexors are evident with full passive combined wrist and finger extension. A platform cast can be applied to improve hand function with or without the thumb enclosed.

Prior to using this cast, the overall tone of the involved extremity must be carefully evaluated. Patients who have relatively mild tone interfering with established muscle control can be considered good candidates.

Effects
1. It can gradually relax the spastic pattern, promoting improved motor function. This inhibitory effect results from the position of the wrist and fingers in the cast.

2. The cast can put the wrist and finger extensors in a position which facilitates active extension.

Contraindications
1. The position of the wrist in extreme extension can cause a carpal tunnel syndrome or circulatory problems.

2. The fingers need to be carefully positioned in the platform. Pressure of the DIP joints secondary to long finger flexor spasticity may cause a boutonniere deformity with hyperextension of the DIP joints and flexion contractures of the PIP joints.

Realistic Goal Setting

Careful assessment of the patient's level of upper extremity function will help you to choose the proper type of cast and establish realistic goals. The patient's ability to activate individual muscles or muscle groups on command will be an indicator for potential outcomes.

A patient with poor voluntary control or a nonfunctional limb may benefit from casting, if only to improve range for hygienic and positioning purposes. The effects of casting may not, in and of themselves, offer prolonged benefits in cases of severe degrees of spasticity. It appears that significant spasticity can recur, especially in the nonfunctional extremity. A maintenance orthosis or bivalved cast would offer a solution to this problem.

For some individuals, casting will only maintain their current range of motion. Since there should be a 5- to 10-degree increase in passive range after removal of each cast, where spasticity is persistent, the results of casting may not be beneficial for increasing range.

Bivalve Casting for Follow-Up Management

For follow-up management, the rigid circular plaster cast can be bivalved to form an anterior and posterior shell. The bivalved cast can be worn as a night and/or day splint to prevent the loss of newly gained range and to prevent further contractures.

There are disadvantages to using plaster for the bivalve cast. The weight of plaster is heavy and offers poor durability. The plaster has a tendency to soften if it gets wet, and it cracks with prolonged use. The plaster also retains body odor. Fiberglass material can be used for increased durability and decreased weight.

Special care must be taken during fabrication of the bivalve cast. The client's arm should be properly positioned in a submaximal range or at the resting posture to avoid improper fit, pressure problems, or pinching of the skin, which in turn will cause difficulty with building up wearing tolerance.

The turnbuckle splint is a double upright long arm orthosis with a turnbuckle on the outside upright. It has a humeral and forearm cuff with velcro straps to provide the control (Figure 274). A patient with moderate to severe spasticity may have pressure area problems with this type of an orthotic device. The arm cuffs must be properly fitting and the pressure equally distributed to prevent skin breakdown. Therapists must carefully evaluate and monitor the use of various orthotic devices. The orthosis should maintain range, provide equalized pressure and proper fit throughout the arm.

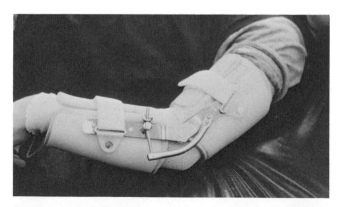

Figure 274

Positioning

Proper positioning of the patient is an important factor to consider prior to casting and throughout the casting program. The effects of improper positioning of the total body, whether in bed or in a wheelchair, can affect the results of the casting program. Support for the shoulder girdle may be a consideration in the more involved extremity, especially in the case of adult hemiparesis. An armrest or lapboard may provide a simple solution. There are commercially available positioning devices and adapted equipment that the therapist and patient can explore.

Relationship of Casting to Neuro-Developmental Treatment

Casting is considered an adjunct to the patient's overall therapy program. The functional goals of the patient should coincide with the goals of the casting program. Ongoing whole-body treatment during the casting series increases the potential benefits. The cast, in position, acts as a third key point of control during mat activities. The therapist can continue to facilitate muscle re-education and muscle strengthening while the spasticity is being reduced.

Phenol Nerve Block

Phenol nerve blocks have been used for the control of spasticity. The phenol temporarily interferes with nerve function, resulting in a decrease in muscle tone. After the phenol nerve block is performed, the patient's arm can be placed into a plaster cast to reverse the contracture. The effects of phenol may last for three to six months. The prolonged benefits of phenol vary in cases of moderate to severe degrees of spasticity. Severe spasticity continues to manifest the original problems of the upper extremity. After the effect of phenol has worn off, those patients with selective motor control appear to maintain or improve in upper extremity function.

Surgery

When conservative methods of casting and standard rehabilitation techniques fail to impact adequately on spasticity, surgical treatment may be investigated. The patient may require surgery to assist with improving cosmesis, hygiene, and function of the upper extremity.

Summary

Patients are carefully evaluated prior to and throughout the casting program. In addition, ongoing monitoring and follow-up are essential for evaluating motor and functional changes. The therapist will decide on the type of cast and follow-up management based on clinical judgment and evaluation skills. Realistic functional goals should be discussed and a program planned and designed to meet the individual needs of the patient. The follow-up management includes careful, detailed instruction to the patient, nursing staff, family, and caregivers. Instructions include proper application and removal, wearing times, precautions, and active use of the extremity during casting.

Case Studies

CASE 1

Mike is a ten-year-old with right hemiplegia, who attends a regular school. Mike wanted his right arm to be "straightened out." A pronation contracture of the forearm in association with a flexion contracture of the elbow limited the active use of the arm to a gross functional assist.

Mike supinated to mid position. He turned his head toward the uninvolved side only. The involved shoulder came forward with the trunk laterally flexed (Figure 275). With bilateral humeral flexion, definite asymmetry in range and head position was noted (Figure 276). The right shoulder girdle was weaker than the left and the scapula was anteriorly tipped, with winging noted on the inferior border.

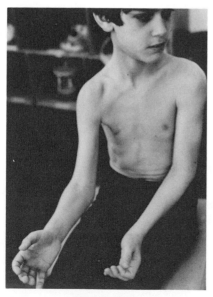

Figure 275

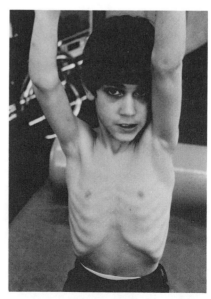

Figure 276

A long arm cast was applied to facilitate the following objectives: (1) increase range in elbow extension and forearm supination, (2) decrease spasticity, (3) improve function, and (4) increase proximal strength. Mike actively worked on a home program of flexing and abducting his right arm through full range to strengthen his shoulder girdle (Figure 277).

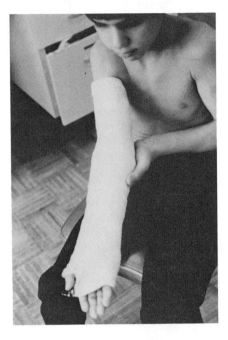

Figure 277

The casting program gradually increased range in forearm supination and elbow extension (Figure 278). The cast provided joint alignment and the external control of spasticity. This allowed him to increase the strength of the shoulder girdle musculature (Figure 279).

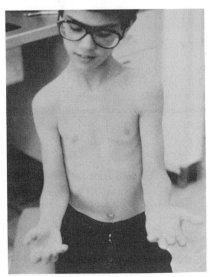

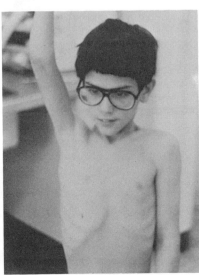

Figure 278   *Figure 279*

Mike's final cast was removed when he acquired full passive supination and elbow extension. To maintain the range gained from the casting program, he wore a bivalved long arm cast whenever he was not involved in therapy or in his home exercise program. Wearing time was gradually decreased to use as a night positioning splint. The new strength and control of the right arm will continue to require monitoring, ongoing evaluation, and night positioning to reinforce the results of casting.

CASE 2

Patty is a nine-year-old with cerebral palsy, spastic quadriplegia. She exhibited mild spasticity in the upper extremities, with the left arm more involved than the right. Passive range of motion in both wrists and fingers were within normal limits.

However, grasp and release were accompanied by wrist flexion. MCP hyperextension was evident with her attempts at wrist extension. Ulnar deviation in the fingers was consistently seen during her primitive grasp and release patterns. In general there was a lack of palmar activity, wrist stability, and digital control (Figure 280).

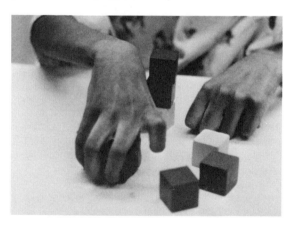

Figure 280

A cast was applied to stabilize the wrist, putting long finger flexors and extensors at an equal advantage. It allowed her to use her fingers with the hand in proper alignment to the forearm. It allowed her to experience grasp and release without MCP hyperextension. During the casting program, Patty worked on her daily self-care skills and tabletop activities requiring grasp and release of various-sized objects (Figure 281).

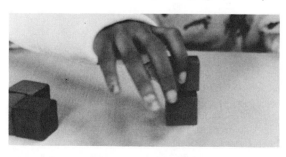

Figure 281

The casting program was followed up with a wrist splint. The splint gave Patty's wrist ongoing support while she continued to develop more mature hand patterns (Figure 282). The current goal of therapy is to help her to develop active wrist stability with palmar activity. When this goal is reached, the wrist support will be discontinued.

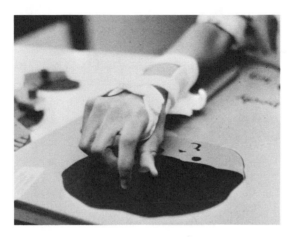

Figure 282

CASE 3

Eleven-year-old Jenny had severe flexion contractures throughout both upper extremities, secondary to anoxia from smoke inhalation. As she became medically stable, an intensive casting program was initiated. Both elbows were casted, one at a time, with humeral enclosed drop-out casts. Each cast was left on between three and five days, depending upon the degree of relaxation of tone and the increase in range. As each elbow dropped out into 10 to 15 degrees of elbow extension, the cast was removed, the skin checked, the arm gently ranged and immediately recasted. As each elbow relaxed to minus 20 degrees of extension, a wrist cast was applied to decrease the wrist flexion contracture. The weight of the wrist cast assisted with a further increase in elbow range. When the elbow and wrist range were complete, a long arm cast was applied to correct the pronation contracture. This was eventually replaced with bivalved positioning splints. The casting program lasted approximately one year during her in-patient stay.

After discharge she was seen as an out-patient for four months and then monitored in a clinic twice a year. Two years post onset, after intensive serial casting, Jenny had functional range in both upper extremities. She was right-hand dominant and demonstrated greater control with her right hand versus the left hand.

Six years post onset, when Jenny was seventeen years old and preparing for college, she returned to occupational therapy. She stated that she was having difficulty in the area of self-care independence because of inadequate pinch in the left hand. Jenny requested a wrist cast for her left hand.

Jenny was seen for a three-week casting program as an out-patient. Her left wrist was generally positioned in flexion, and ulnar deviation and spasticity were noted in the thenar and hypothenar eminence. These problems with tone and alignment resulted in a lateral pinch. She demonstrated difficulty actively using her thumb for a fingertip pinch.

The first wrist cast was left on for one week to align the wrist in neutral. After it was removed, she was better able to actively oppose thumb to index finger but continued to be influenced by flexion/adduction spasticity. Jenny did not have full active range of thumb extension and abduction. She hyperextended at the IP and MCP joints of the thumb to compensate for her limitations in range (Figure 283).

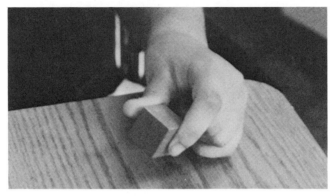

Figure 283

The second wrist cast enclosed the thumb and positioned it in extension with the wrist maintained in neutral. This position assisted with decreasing the tightness of the hand (Figure 284). After removal of the cast, the thumb appeared more relaxed. Opposition was much easier to perform (Figure 285). However, Jenny continued to demonstrate difficulty with wrist extension during active prehension. Her final cast aligned the thumb in slight abduction/opposition with the wrist positioned in extension (Figure 286).

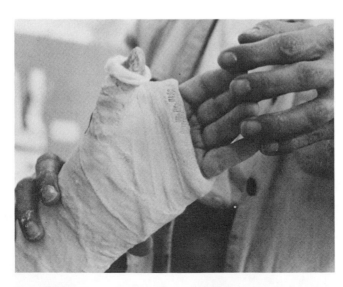

Figure 284

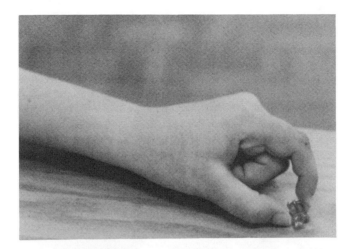

Figure 285

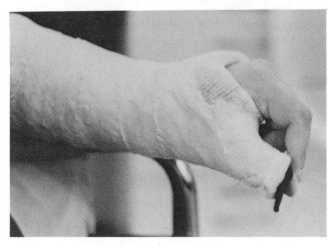

Figure 286

Functionally, Jenny's prehension pattern improved by aligning the joints and decreasing the tone. However, habitual use of the lateral pinch before casting made it a difficult pattern to change. When stressed, Jenny returned to her original prehension pattern (Figure 287).

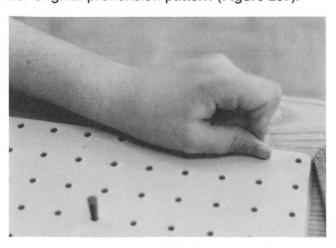

Figure 287

A night splint was fabricated to maintain the range and alignment of the thumb and wrist (Figure 288). A wrist splint was fabricated for day wear. The wrist splint provided stability and alignment at the wrist for a stronger pinch and other prehension patterns. Without the use of the splint, she had difficulty controlling the alignment of wrist and thumb during function (Figure 289). After the three-week out-patient casting program, Jenny was admitted into a rehabilitation facility. Her personal goals were to upgrade activities of daily living skills prior to college.

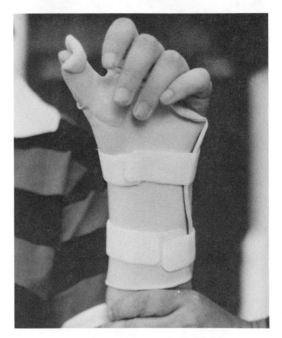

Figure 288

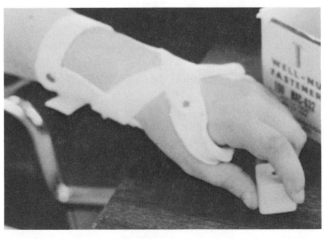

Figure 289

The effects of casting on function must be assessed repeatedly with the patient in a variety of functional situations. Continued monitoring of the client is essential prior to and after the casting program. The motivation and cognitive level of the patient will positively impact on the casting program and follow-up.

Bibliography for Appendix B

Bankov, S. 1975. A test for differentiation between contracture and spasm of the biceps muscle in post traumatic rigidities of the elbow joint. *The Hand* 7:263-265.

Bell, J. 1978. Plaster cylinder casting of contractures of interphalangeal joints. In *The rehabilitation of the hand,* edited by Hunter, Schneider, Mackin, and Bell. St. Louis, MO: C.V. Mosby Co.

———. 1985a. Plaster casting of the remodeling of soft tissue: Part II. *The Star* 44:10-16.

Bishop, B. 1977. Spasticity: Its physiology and management, Parts I-IV. *Physical Therapy* 57:371-401.

Bobath, B. 1978. *Adult hemiplegia: Evaluation and treatment.* London: William Heinemann Medical Books, Ltd.

Booth, B. J., M. Doyle, and J. Montgomery. 1983. Serial casting for the management of spasticity in the head-injured adult. *Physical Therapy* 63:1960-1966.

Braun, R. M., M. Hoffer, V. Mooney. 1973. Phenol nerve block in the treatment of acquired spastic hemiplegia in the upper limb. *Journal of Bone and Joint Surgery* 55A:580-585.

Brodal, P. 1981. *Neurological anatomy in relation to clinical medicine.* New York: Oxford University Press.

Caldwell, C., and R. Braun. 1974. Spasticity in the upper extremity. *Clinical Orthopaedics and Related Research* 104:80-94.

Cherry, D. 1980. Review of physical therapy alternatives for reducing muscle contracture. *Physical Therapy* 60:877-881.

Crutchfield, C., and M. Barnes. 1974. *The neurophysiological bases of patient treatment.* Vol. 1: *The muscle spindle.* Atlanta, GA: Stokesville Publishing Co.

Edstrom, L. 1970. Selective changes in the sizes of red and white muscle fibres in upper motor lesions and parkinsonism. *Journal of the Neurological Sciences* (Netherlands) 2:537-550.

Freehafer, A. 1977. Flexion and supination deformities of the elbow in tetraplegia. *Paraplegia* 15:221-225.

Garland, D., R. Thompson, and R. Waters. 1980. Musculocutaneous neurectomy for spastic elbow flexion in non-functional upper extremities in adults. *Journal of Bone and Joint Surgery* 62:108-112.

Garland, D., L. Menachem, and M. Keenan. 1984. Percutaneous phenol blocks to motor points of spastic forearm muscles in head injured adults. *Archives of Physical Medicine and Rehabilitation* 65:243-244.

King, T. 1982. Plaster splinting as a means of reducing elbow flexor spasticity: A case study. *American Journal of Occupational Therapy* 36:671-673.

Kozole, K., and A. Yasukawa. 1982. An extension orthosis for the management of elbow flexion contractures. *Journal of Orthotics and Prosthetics* 82:50-62.

McCollough, N. 1978. Orthotic management in adult hemiplegia. *Clinical Orthopaedics and Related Research* 131:38-40.

Mills, V. 1984. Electromyographic results of inhibitory splinting. *Physical Therapy* 64:190-193.

Mital, M. 1979. Lengthening of the elbow flexors in cerebral palsy. *Journal of Bone and Joint Surgery* 61A:515-522.

Professional Staff Association of Rancho Los Amigos Hospital. 1979. *Rehabilitation of the head injured adult.* Downey, CA: Rancho Los Amigos Hospital.

Williams, P., and G. Goldspink. 1978. Changes in sarcomere length and physiological properties in immobilized muscles. *Journal of Anatomy* 127:459-468.

Wood, K. 1978. The use of phenol as a neurolytic agent: A review. *Pain* 5:205-229.

About the Authors of Appendix B

Audrey Yasukawa received her masters degree in occupational therapy from Western Michigan University in 1978. She is currently employed at LaRabida Children's Hospital and has lectured nationally on topics related to occupational therapy. Audrey is certified in adult hemiplegia and pediatric neurodevelopmental treatment. She resides in Chicago.

Judy Hill holds a B.S. degree in occupational therapy from the University of Wisconsin at Madison. She is a clinical specialist at the Rehabilitation Institute of Chicago and is certified in neurodevelopmental treatment for adult hemiplegia. Judy was an editor and contributing author for *Spinal cord injury: A guide to functional outcomes in occupational therapy.* Judy has lectured nationally on inhibitory casting of the upper extremities.

A *Kinesiological Analysis* of *Dynamic Sitting*

Barbara Hypes, P.T.

Introduction

When attending to upper extremity function, it is valuable to understand the components of a dynamically stable sitting base. This means that we can sit relatively still during upper extremity function, while we shift our body weight to reach. Dynamic sitting is accomplished by muscles that connect the trunk to the pelvis as well as muscles that connect the pelvis to the legs.

The Pelvis in Sitting

The pelvis is in a neutral position when the two bony prominences at the front of the pelvis (anterior superior iliac spine and the pubic symphysis) are in the same vertical plane (Kendall and McCreary 1982) (Figure 290). For the pelvis to be level, the two anterior superior iliac spines should be in the same horizontal plane.

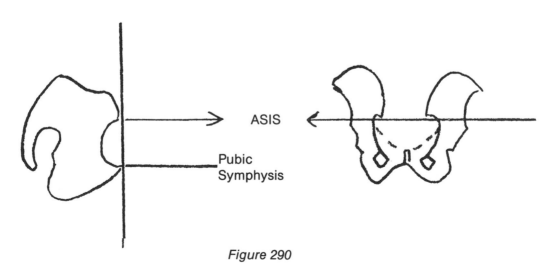

ASIS

Pubic
Symphysis

Figure 290

SPINAL EXTENSORS

Posteriorly, the spinal extensors connect the bony prominences of the vertebra to surrounding vertebra. Collectively, they connect the back of the skull to the posterior iliac crest and sacrum (Figure 291). Unopposed contraction of the spinal extensors will bring the head closer to the sacrum. In our patients we see this as generalized hyperextension. The pelvis is pulled into an anterior tilt and the ribs are forced to flare (Figure 292).

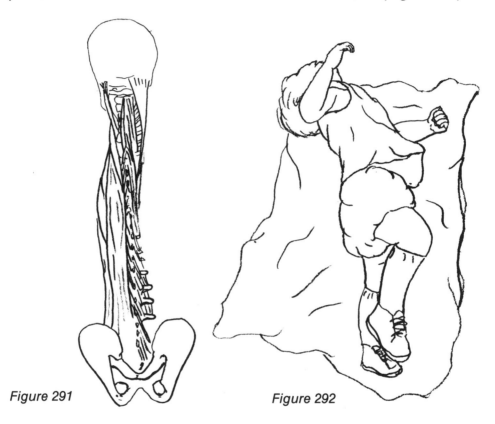

Figure 291

Figure 292

RECTUS ABDOMINUS

One muscle that provides an anterior connection between pelvis and trunk, is the rectus abdominus (Figure 293). This muscle originates on the fifth, sixth, and seventh ribs and the xiphoid process of the sternum. It inserts onto the pubic crest and symphysis. When this muscle works, it holds the upper and lower body together anteriorly. The pubic symphysis and sternum are pulled closer together. This action mechanically pulls the pelvis into a posterior tilt and allows the seventh through the twelfth ribs to flare laterally (Figure 294). This may provide a patient with enough stability to support hip flexor activity. However, it does not provide a base for lateral or posterior control.

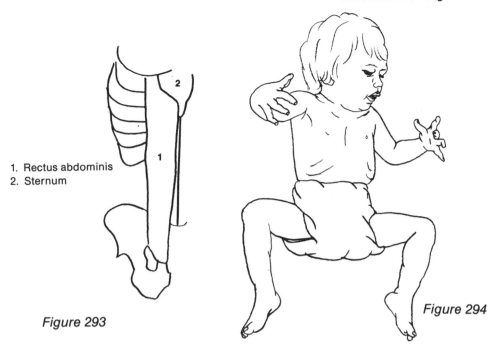

1. Rectus abdominis
2. Sternum

Figure 293

Figure 294

Unopposed use of either the spinal extensors or rectus abdominus provides only limited control around the trunk, pulling the pelvis out of an efficient alignment. Therefore, the spinal extensors and rectus abdominus must work cooperatively to align the pelvis on the trunk in an anterior and posterior plane. In addition, the pelvis needs stability in lateral and diagonal planes. This is provided by the abdominal obliques.

ABDOMINAL OBLIQUES

The abdominal obliques consist of three interwoven muscles. These muscles are the external oblique, internal oblique, and transverse abdominus.

The external obliques originate from ribs five through twelve, intertwining with the serratus anterior and the latissimus dorsi (Figure 295). The anterior fibers insert into the broad, flat aponeurosis of the linea alba. The lateral fibers insert onto the anterior portion of the pelvis. With the two sides of the external oblique acting together, the trunk moves closer to the pelvis, anteriorly (Figure 296). When the pelvis is stabilized and one side is acting alone, the direction of the movement will be diagonal. For example, the anterior fibers of the right external oblique will pull the right trunk closer to the left side of the pelvis (Figure 297). On the other hand, when the trunk is stabilized, the right anterior oblique fibers will pull the left pelvis closer to the right side of the trunk (see Figure 300).

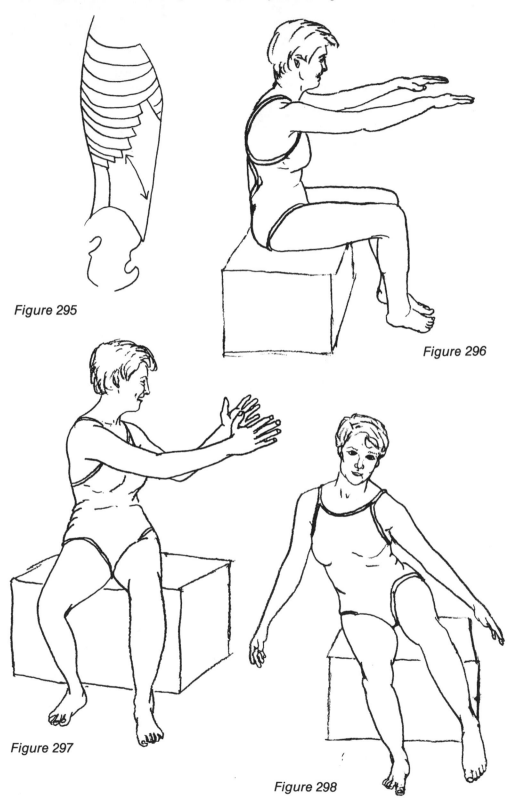

Figure 295

Figure 296

Figure 297

Figure 298

The lateral fibers of the external obliques have a strong influence on the lumbar spine. Acting bilaterally, they bring the pelvis into a posterior tilt, causing the lumbar spine to flatten. Acting unilaterally, these fibers laterally flex the trunk, bringing the ribs and pelvis closer together (Figure 298). The external oblique muscle fibers angle downward from the ribs toward the umbilicus and work in conjunction with the internal oblique fibers.

The internal oblique has a lower, anterior portion as well as a lateral portion (Figure 299). These fibers collectively arise from the inguinal ligament, iliac crest, and thoracolumbar fascia. The anterior fibers insert into the linea alba via the aponeurosis and onto the pubic crest. The lateral fibers angle from the iliac crest diagonally forward and up to insert on the tenth to twelfth ribs as well as the aponeurosis.

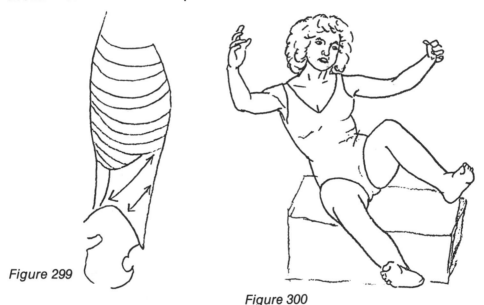

Figure 299

Figure 300

Acting bilaterally, the internal oblique fibers bring the trunk and pelvis closer together, as in Figure 296. Unilaterally the anterior fibers of the internal obliques on the right work with the anterior fibers of the external obliques on the left. When the trunk is stabilized, these muscles pull the left side of the pelvis toward the right lower ribs (Figure 300). When the pelvis is stabilized, these muscles pull the right lower ribs toward the left side of the pelvis, as in Figure 297. Acting unilaterally, the lateral fibers of the internal oblique on the right side act with the lateral fibers of the external oblique on the right side to laterally flex trunk and pelvis, as in Figure 298.

The internal and external obliques work together to move the trunk diagonally on a stable pelvis. For example, when the patient bears weight on the right hip and the right ribs are pulled closer to the left pelvis, this reflects flexion with rotation (see Figure 300). We commonly refer to this as an equilibrium reaction. When these same muscles are acting with the patient's weight on the left hip, this reflects extension with rotation (Figure 301). We commonly refer to this as a protective reaction.

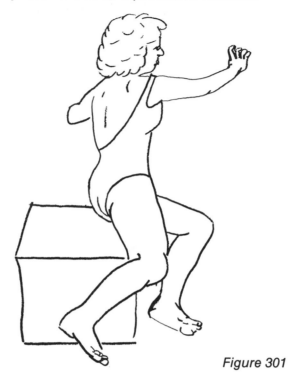

Figure 301

The third muscle in the oblique group is the transverse abdominis. This muscle originates from the last six ribs and anterior three-fourths of the iliac crest. It intertwines with the diaphragm, the thoracolumbar fascia, and the inguinal ligament. These fibers insert into the linea alba and pubic crest via the aponeurosis. Dynamically the transverse abdominus acts to enclose the abdominal viscera and stabilize the linea alba while the external and internal obliques flex the trunk.

LATISSIMUS DORSI

The latissimus dorsi (Figure 302) originates from the last six thoracic vertebrae, last four ribs, from the thoracolumbar fascia of the lumbar and sacral vertebrae, from the posterior third of the iliac crest, and a slip from the inferior angle of the scapula. These fibers insert on the intertubercular groove of the humerus. Therefore, this muscle connects the humerus to the pelvis.

Acting unilaterally with a fixed origin, the muscle will internally rotate, adduct and extend the humerus, depress the shoulder girdle, and laterally flex the trunk (Figure 303). Acting unilaterally with a fixed insertion, the muscle will pull the pelvis anteriorly and laterally (Figure 304). Acting bilaterally, the fibers hyperextend the spine and tilt the pelvis anteriorly (Figure 305).

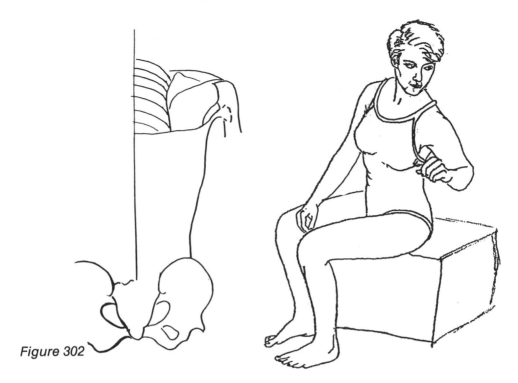

Figure 302

Figure 303

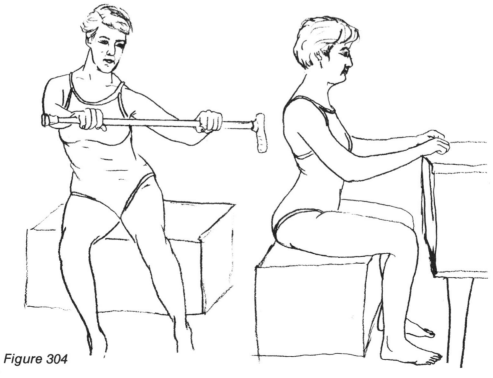

Figure 304

Figure 305

In sacral sitting, where the center of gravity is behind the hips, this muscle, acting bilaterally, will flex the trunk into gravity (Figure 306). When the center of gravity is in front of the axis of motion in sitting, the latissimus dorsi, acting bilaterally, will pull the lumbar spine into a lordosis with an anterior tilt of the pelvis as in Figure 305.

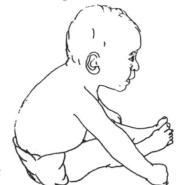

Figure 306

A third possibility in sitting is seen when the muscle acts unilaterally, flexing one side of the body into gravity, hiking the pelvis up, and pulling the shoulder and humerus down as in Figure 303. This lateral flexion into gravity is also seen in stance and gait, with the pelvis anteriorly and laterally tipped. Because it elevates the pelvis, the patient may appear to have a leg length discrepancy (Figure 307). Use of plantar flexion in all phases of gait will make this shortened side functionally longer. This posture also puts the patient at risk for scoliosis since the spine follows the anterior and lateral movement of the pelvis.

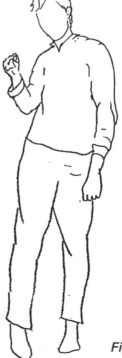

Figure 307

Hip Flexors

ILIOPSOAS

The iliopsoas is formed by the psoas major, psoas minor, and iliacus (Figure 308). The origin of the psoas muscle is on the ventral surface of the transverse processes of the lumbar vertebrae. It inserts on the lesser trochanter of the femur. The iliacus origin is from the iliac fossa and internal lip of the iliac crest. The fibers insert into the tendon of the psoas major. Together this group acts as a one-joint muscle across the hip.

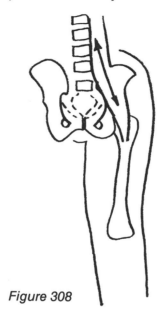

Figure 308

With the origin stabilized, the iliopsoas acts to flex the femur on the trunk (Figure 309). With the insertion stabilized, the muscle acting bilaterally will flex a stable trunk over the femurs as in a sit-up performed when the feet

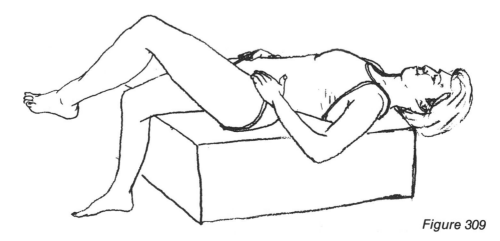

Figure 309

are stabilized (Figure 310). Sit-ups are frequently performed in this fashion with the intent of strengthening abdominal obliques. It is worth emphasizing that hip flexors are being strengthened in this type of sit-up.

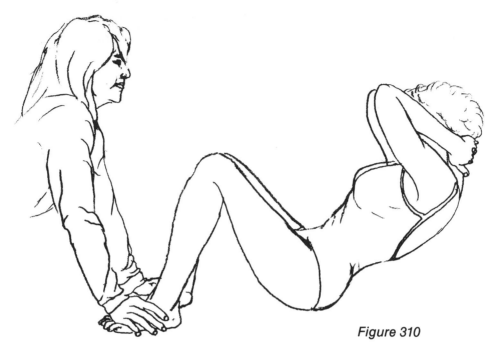

Figure 310

When the iliopsoas bilaterally acts unopposed, it moves the lumbar spine closer to the femurs. This action will cause a lordosis when the pelvis is in front of the hips as in Figure 305. In sacral sitting, where the pelvis is behind the hips, the patient can hold this position using hip flexors as in Figure 306.

RECTUS FEMORIS

The rectus femoris (Figure 311) is one of four muscles that comprise the quadriceps femoris muscle group. This muscle originates from the anterior inferior iliac spine and groove above the acetabulum. It inserts with the other three muscles on the proximal border of the patella, through the patellar ligament to the tuberosity of the tibia.

The rectus femoris can act to extend the knee joint and flex the hip. When this two-joint muscle is contracted, the patient may look fine in standing, with only one joint on stretch. But in kneeling, with the rectus femoris on stretch across the hip and the knee, the patient may demonstrate an anterior pelvic tilt (Figure 312). Since the insertion of the muscle is stable against the weight-bearing surface in kneeling, the origin pulls the pelvis forward.

The function of the quadriceps femoris group is primarily for knee extension. Weakness in this muscle group interferes with stair climbing and the ability to move up and down from sitting.

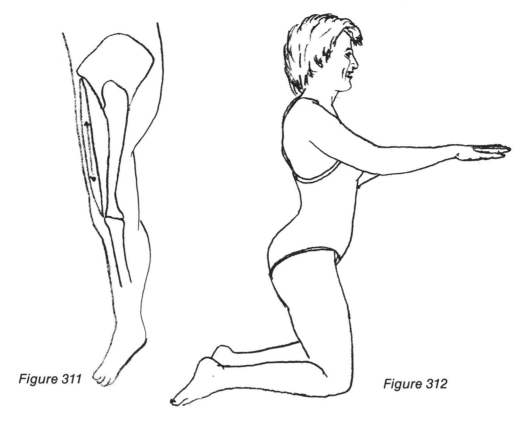

Figure 311

Figure 312

Hip Extensors

GLUTEUS MAXIMUS

The gluteus maximus originates from the ilium, lower part of the sacrum and coccyx, and aponeurosis of the erector spinae (Figure 313). It inserts into the iliotibial tract of the fascia latae and onto the femur. This muscle acts as a primary extensor of the femur on the pelvis. When the pelvis is stabilized with the patient in prone, this muscle will lift the femur off the surface.

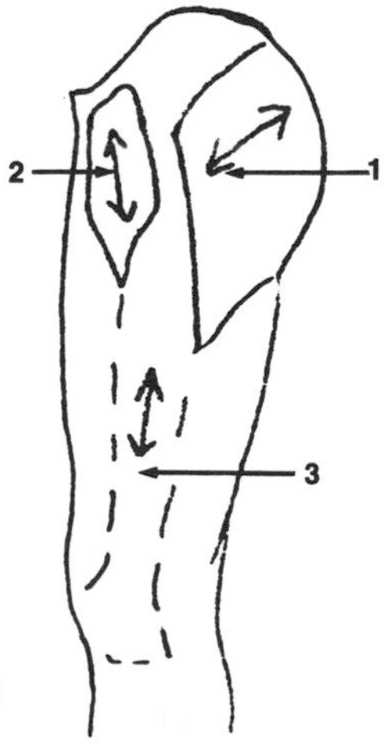

1. Gluteus maximus
2. Tensor fascia latae
3. Iliotibial band

Figure 313

In sitting, the gluteus maximus work dynamically against the surface. Further, they work eccentrically to allow the patient to bend forward for reach. They work concentrically to return the upper body to the upright. The upper half of the body moves over the lower half, with pelvis riding over hips (Figure 314). Adequate length of the proximal end of the hamstrings is needed for this movement of the pelvis over the femurs.

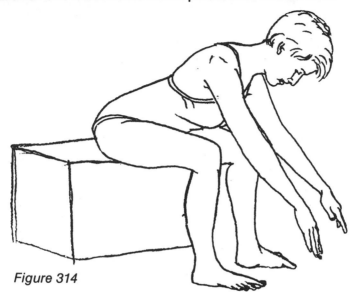

Figure 314

Hamstrings

The hamstrings include the semitendinosus, semimembranosus, and the biceps femoris (Figure 315). These muscles originate from the tuberosity of the ischium. They insert on the medial and lateral condyles of the tibia and the head of the fibula. These muscles flex the knee and, because of their pelvic attachment, they can extend the femur on the pelvis.

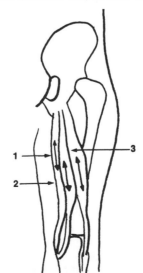

1. Biceps femoris
2. Semitendinosus
3. Semimembranosus

Figure 315

Acting unopposed with a stabilized origin, the hamstrings flex the knees and extend the hips. In long sitting with the pelvis stabilized in neutral and limited hamstring length, the knee will bend (Figure 316). If the knees are stabilized, the pelvis will be pulled posteriorly and the lumbar spine will flatten (Figure 317). Children with limited hamstring length may opt for W-sitting on the floor since the position of the legs allows for less pull on this muscle.

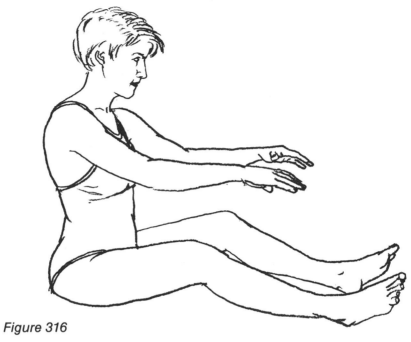

Figure 316

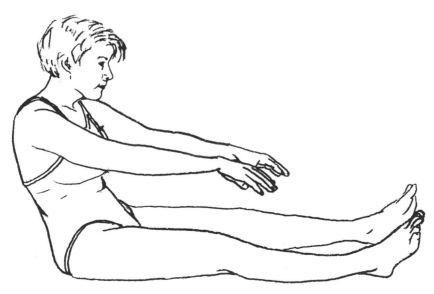

Figure 317

Hip Abduction

GLUTEUS MEDIUS

The gluteus medius is a primary hip abductor (Figure 318). This muscle originates from the external surface of the ilium. It inserts on the greater

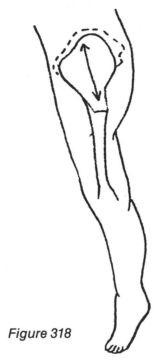

Figure 318

trochanter of the femur. When the trunk is stabilized in sidelying, this muscle lifts the femur laterally toward the pelvis (Figure 319).

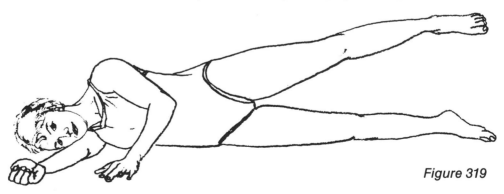

Figure 319

Weakness in the gluteus medius provides a poor base for reach in sitting. When we reach toward the sides, our legs stabilize onto the supporting surface through the action of hip abduction and extension. When hip abductors are weak, the patient will laterally flex on the weight-bearing side (Figure 320). This will serve to flex the upper torso into gravity. This pattern of movement interferes with controlled weight shifts and prevents righting and equilibrium reactions.

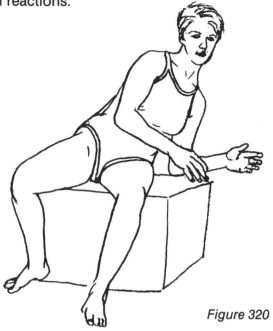

Figure 320

TENSOR FASCIA LATAE

This muscle originates from the anterior lip of the iliac crest and the anterior superior iliac spine (refer to Figure 313). It inserts into the iliotibial tract of the fascia latae.

The tensor fascia latae flexes, internally rotates, and abducts the femur on the pelvis. This muscle may be shortened in patients that demonstrate more primitive hip control. In sitting and prone, the patient may stabilize into the surface with hip flexion, abduction, and external rotation (Figure 321). It is this position that allows shortening of this muscle.

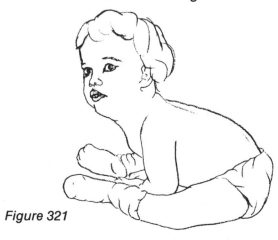

Figure 321

Hip Adduction

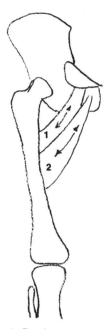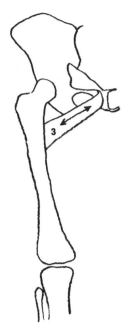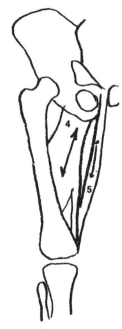

1. Pectineus
2. Adductor longus

3. Adductor brevis

4. Adductor magnus
5. Gracilis

Figure 322

PECTINEUS

The hip adductors consist of a group of five muscles. The pectineus originates on the pubic surface of the pelvis and inserts on the pectineal line of the femur. This muscle adducts the femur, approximating the femur to the pubic portion of the pelvis. It can also assist in flexion of the hip joint due to its pelvic origin.

ADDUCTOR MAGNUS

The adductor magnus originates from the inferior portion of the pubic and ischial surface and from the ishial tuberosity. It inserts throughout the medial shaft of the femur. These attachments make this muscle a very powerful adductor. The anterior attachments on the pubic and ischial surfaces allow this muscle to assist in hip flexion, whereas the attachment on the ischial tuberiosity allow the muscle to assist in hip extension.

GRACILIS

The gracilis originates from the inferior border of the pubic surface and inserts on the medial surface of the tibia. In addition to adducting the hip joint, this muscle can also flex and medially rotate the knee joint.

ADDUCTOR BREVIS

The adductor brevis originates from the inferior surface of the pubis and inserts on the pectineal line of the femur. This muscle can adduct the femur and assist in hip flexion.

ADDUCTOR LONGUS

The adductor longus originates from the anterior surface of the pubis and inserts into the linear aspect of the femur. This muscle can adduct the femur and assist in hip flexion.

Since the adductors originate on the pelvis from the pubic symphysis to the ischial tuberosity, they can effect both medial and lateral rotation of the hip joint dependent on the mechanical axis of motion of the hip joint. This axis can be altered by the position of the pelvis and the action of other muscles stabilizing the trunk, pelvis, and femur. During true adduction, this group of muscles would not act as either medial or lateral rotators of the hip.

True adduction of the hip joint is tested in sidelying. The examiner holds the upper leg. The patient should stabilize the upper body, then bring the lower leg up from the table without rotation, hip flexion, hip extension, or tilting of the pelvis (Figure 323).

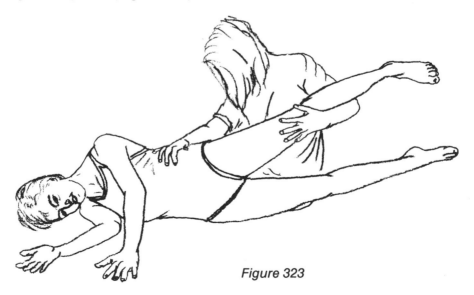

Figure 323

A posterior pelvic tilt with hip extension allows substitution with the lower fibers of the gluteus maximus (Figure 324). An anterior tilt with hip flexion

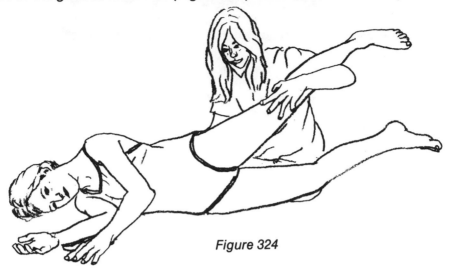

Figure 324

allows substitution with the hip flexors (Figure 325). Remember, the adductor longus, adductor brevis, and pectineus can assist in hip flexion. Consequently, hip flexion with adduction may demonstrate that these adductors are more active than the other adductors. On the other hand, it may demonstrate that the hip extensors are not helping to keep the femur in a neutral position.

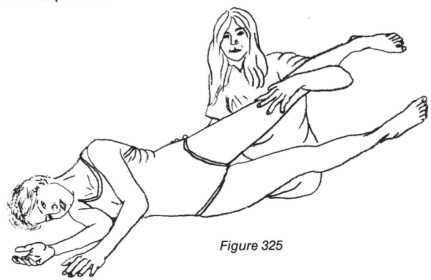

Figure 325

Shortness in the hip adductors laterally displaces the pelvis. This causes the pelvis on the side of the contracture to be raised in stance (Figure 326). Therefore the patient must make the extremity longer on that side by plantar flexing the ankle. In sitting, this tightness causes posterior displacement of the pelvis on the contracted side (Figure 327) or adduction of the femur if the pelvis is stabilized.

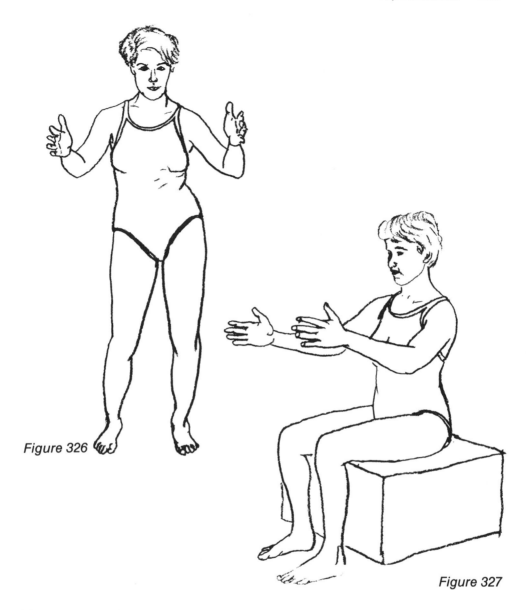

Figure 326

Figure 327

Normally in sitting, the adductors stabilize the femurs on the pelvis medially and work synergistically with the other hip muscles. This gives the patient freedom to turn and reach in any direction.

If the patient sits in hip flexion, the adductors help to stabilize them into gravity. When the patient is in an anterior tilt with hyperflexion in the hips, the adductors push into the surface for stability. The extreme of this position is W-sitting with an anterior pelvic tilt. When the patient sits on the sacrum, forcing the pelvis into a posterior pelvic tilt, the rectus abdominus stabilizes the trunk to the pubis while three of the adductors stabilize the legs to the pubis.

Since the mechanical axis of motion of the hips is altered by the alignment of the pelvis in both of these positions, the adductors also function as medial rotators. Therefore a strong pattern of hip flexion, adduction, and internal rotation develops (Figure 328). In either an anterior or a posterior pelvic tilt, the patient can only move into flexion or extension with control. They cannot control lateral or diagonal weight shifting.

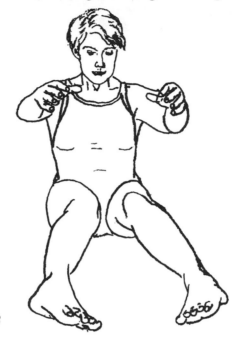

Figure 328

Dynamic Interaction of Muscles in Sitting

Many muscles attach to the pelvis from the spine, ribs, and femurs. To maintain the neutral pelvic alignment, these muscles must work together. The obliques, together with the rectus abdominus, latissimus dorsi, and spinal extensors, form a girdle connecting the trunk and the pelvis. When these muscles work together, they provide stability to the ribs and abdominal walls. They assist the diaphragm in respiration by supporting the sternum and rib cage. In addition, they provide a stable trunk for upper extremity function.

Dynamically, this group of muscles allows the trunk to move in any direction on a stable pelvis. They allow the pelvis to move on a stable trunk. Collectively, they control upper body rotation on a stable lower body and vice versa.

While trunk control neutralizes the pelvis, hip control maintains the alignment of pelvis over the hips. Consequently, the lower extremities stabilize the body against the surface in sitting, allowing freedom of the arms for function.

Reach beyond the length of the arm requires a weight shift. Weight shift requires an interplay between trunk and hip muscles. For example, reach with a lateral weight shift will require lateral flexion on the non-weight-bearing side and active hips against the surface on the weight-bearing side. The anterior, posterior control utilized when taking off a T-shirt will require trunk flexion and extension with hips working against the surface. The diagonal control necessary for lower-body dressing will require movement of one shoulder to the opposite pelvis, or flexion with rotation in the trunk. The weight bearing hip works against the surface allowing the non-weight-bearing femur to move off the stable pelvis.

Summary

When treating the neurologically impaired patient, we are treating the whole body. All of the parts are connected. A problem in one area can create problems in other areas of the body. The pelvis is a central part of this whole. Muscle activity connecting ribs and spine to the pelvis and the pelvis to the femurs will impact significantly on upper extremity function.

Reference

Kendall, F., and E. McCreary. 1982. *Muscle testing and function.* Baltimore, MD: Williams and Wilkins.

Additional Readings

Anderson, T. 1976. *Grant's atlas of anatomy.* 7th ed. Baltimore, MD: The Williams and Wilkins Co.

Hollingshead, W. 1976. *Functional anatomy of the limbs and back.* 4th ed. Philadelpia, PA: W.B. Saunders, Co.

Hoppenfield, S. 1976. *Physical examination of the spine and extremities.* New York: Appleton-Centruy-Crofts.

Kapandji, I. 1974. *The physiology of the joints,* Vol. 3. New York: Churchill Livingstone.

McMinn, R., and R. Hutchings. 1977. *Color atlas of human anatomy.* Chicago, IL: Medical Publishers, Inc.

Sieg, K., and S. Adams. 1985. *Illustrated essentials of musculoskeletal anatomy.* 2nd ed. Gainesville, FL: Megabooks.

About the Author of Appendix C

Barbara Hypes recieved her B.S. degree in physical therapy at Indiana University/Purdue University in Indianapolis. She is certified in neurodevelopmental treatment and lectures throughout the United States on topics related to the treatment of cerebral palsy. She maintains a private practice in the Milwaukee area.

More valuable resources from Regi Boehme, OTR . . .

APPROACH TO TREATMENT OF THE BABY (Revised 1990); This easy-to-use manual gives you a detailed look at the abnormal baby—with a focus on cerebral palsy. Bobath and NDT approaches are included in the illustrated treatment rationale. Drawings cover elongation of the trunk, rectus abdominis, hip flexors; lumbar extension; maximum loading of upper extremities; and much more.

Catalog No. 4218-Y   **$15**

DEVELOPING MID-RANGE CONTROL AND FUNCTION in Children with Fluctuat-ing Muscle Tone (Revised 1990)

This resource gives you an easy-to-understand overview of the athetoid child. You'll have clear drawings of both conditions and treatment techniques, with complete descriptions. Topics cover principles of neuro-developmental treatment, classification of types according to quality of fluctuating postural tone, suggested readings, and much more!

Catalog No. 4219-Y   **$15**

THE HYPOTONIC CHILD—Treatment for Postural Control, Endurance, Strength, and Sensory Organization (Revised 1990)

This resource gives you practical information and clear illustrations for treatment of the hypotonic child. You'll have an overview of basic problems including early signs, quality of tone, consequences, postural instability, hypermobility, possible deformities, respiration, and much more!

Catalog No. 4220-Y   **$15**

More important materials from Therapy Skill Builders . . .

DEVELOPMENTAL POSITION STICKERS (1987)
by Marsha Dunn Klein, M.Ed., O.T.R.

These illustrated stickers present 25 neurodevelopmental positions frequently recommended by occupational therapists to help physically handicapped children or adults at work, rest, and play. Active, sitting, and carrying positions are featured.

Catalog No. 7428-Y   **$16.95**

FEEDING POSITION STICKERS (1987)   *by Marsha Dunn Klein, M.Ed., O.T.R.*

Here are stick-on pictures that illustrate 13 positions recommended to help physically handicapped children maximize oral motor skills for eating.

Catalog No. 7440-Y   **$11.95**

BABY POSITION STICKERS (1987)
by Marsha Dunn Klein, M.Ed., O.T.R., and Nancy J. Harris, O.T.R.

The 31 illustrations on these stickers show positions to facilitate normalized developmental movement patterns in babies up to 18 months old.

Catalog No. 7436-Y   **$18.95**

NEONATAL POSITION STICKERS (1987)
by Marsha Dunn Klein, M.Ed., O.T.R., and Nancy J. Harris, O.T.R.

These illustrated stickers offer 21 positions to facilitate normalized developmental movement patterns in high-risk newborns. These methods of handling, positioning, feeding, and interacting can be used in education of parents and medical staff . . . and can make the transition from hospital to home a positive experience for both baby and caregiver.

Catalog No. 7471-Y   **$14.95**

PRE-FEEDING SKILLS (1987)
by Suzanne Evans Morris, Ph.D., CCC-SLP, and Marsha Dunn Klein, M.Ed., O.T.R.

Here's a problem-solving approach to remediating oral-motor disorders. This resource includes comprehensive information from anatomy and normal development to assessment and treatment. It includes 52 Participation Experiences giving you the opportunity to be an active participant in learning, plus more than 550 illustrations and in-depth information on adaptive pre-feeding materials.

Catalog No. 7406-Y   **$49**

Therapy Skill Builders
A division of
Communication Skill Builders ®
3830 E. Bellevue/P.O. Box 42050
Tucson, Arizona 85733/(602) 323-7500